RESPIRATORY NURSING CARE
Physiology and Technique

880 1325 3172

16   1193

RESPIRATORY NURSING CARE
Physiology and Technique

Jacqueline F. Wade, R.N., S.C.M., B.T.A.

Pulmonary Research Associate, Sequoia District Hospital,
Redwood City, California; formerly Senior Pulmonary Function
Technician and Staff Nurse in Intensive Care,
Stanford University Medical Center,
Stanford, California

SECOND EDITION

with 51 *illustrations*

The C. V. Mosby Company

Saint Louis   1977

SECOND EDITION

Copyright © 1977 by The C. V. Mosby Company

All rights reserved. No part of this book may be reproduced in
any manner without written permission of the publisher.

Previous edition copyrighted 1973

Printed in the United States of America

The C. V. Mosby Company
11830 Westline Industrial Drive, St. Louis, Missouri 63141

Library of Congress Cataloging in Publication Data

Wade, Jacqueline F   1939-
    Respiratory nursing care.

    Bibliography: p.
    Includes index.
    1. Respiratory disease nursing.   2. Respiratory or-
gans.   I. Title.
RC735.5.W3   1977   612′.2′024613   76-55741
ISBN 0-8016-5281-2

TS/VH/VH 9 8 7 6 5 4 3 2

To
Bill
and
Rebecca Anne

PREFACE

With advances in medical technology, patient care becomes more sophisticated, and a nurse's role stretches far beyond the demands of pure nursing; however, Florence Nightingale's philosophy that a patient should come to no harm is most applicable to these times. This places the nurse as guardian, protector, decision-maker, and educator, but most of all a professional practitioner. In no area of nursing is this philosophy put to the test more than in respiratory care.

As more specialty areas evolve, we tend to isolate ourselves within our specialty. The patient then becomes just another "heart," "neuro," "renal," and so on. But most patients—from the elderly gentleman recovering from a herniorrhaphy to the young man in an automobile accident—need respiratory care. This means that whatever area of nursing we choose, we must know how to protect our patients from respiratory complications, know what factors may predispose them to such problems, and understand methods of management.

The second edition is expanded to further the philosophy that a working knowledge of respiratory physiology is essential to respiratory nursing care. Emphasis is again placed on application of physiology and nursing therapy to prevent respiratory complications. With these ideas in mind, a new chapter on bedside monitoring has been added. Also included are new sections on chest physical assessment and interpretation of chest x-ray films.

I wish to thank Dr. Bernhard A. Votteri, Director of Critical Care at Sequoia District Hospital, for his continued support during the preparation of this revision and also for taking time from his duties to read the manuscript and make helpful suggestions. My thanks also go to the ICU nurses and respiratory therapists at Sequoia who were always willing to answer questions and let me barge in during procedures.

I am grateful to Lee Holt for his new illustrations and to Karen Jamison for a professional job of typing the manuscript.

Jacqueline F. Wade

CONTENTS

RESPIRATORY NURSING CARE
Physiology and Technique

1 / PHYSIOLOGY AND BIOLOGY OF RESPIRATION

For life to continue, the human body must receive oxygen and give up carbon dioxide. This process is known as respiration and is accomplished through the inter-relationship of many systems.

Respiration is generally thought of as the process of gas exchange within the lungs, the *physiologic* aspect; but respiration also occurs in the *biologic* sense at the cellular level, where oxygen is used in oxidative tissue metabolism and carbon dioxide is eliminated as a waste product of such metabolism.

This chapter is designed to give the nurse a series of physiologic and biologic links in the process of respiration. The emphasis is on pulmonary microstructure with only a brief overview of gross anatomy. More detailed accounts can be found in the many volumes devoted to this subject.

PHYSIOLOGY OF RESPIRATION
Respiratory tract

The respiratory tract is divided into upper and lower portions and is a series of conducting passageways that begins at the nose and terminates at the alveolar surface. The upper respiratory tract is made up of the nose, pharynx, and larynx. Its functions include the preparation of inspired air for entry into the lungs, which is accomplished through filtration, humidification, and heat supply.

Filtration of particles of dust, dirt, and bacteria occurs mainly in the nasal passages. This process of the upper respiratory tract is so important that special attention is given to it on p. 10.

Air is warmed and moistened as it passes through the entire respiratory tract, but the greatest percentage of humidification occurs in the nose. When the respiratory tract is bypassed, as with tracheostomy, the replacement of the air conditioning functions of the nose by artificial means is vital.

Trachea and bronchi. The trachea is approximately 5 inches long with an average diameter of 1 inch. It is essentially a midline structure and is composed of smooth muscle with regularly placed cartilaginous rings that are horseshoe shaped and incomplete posteriorly. A membranous sheath forms the flat, posterior portion of the trachea, which lies close to the esophagus.

At its lower end (carina) the trachea divides into the right and left main bronchi.

1

The right main bronchus extends as a shorter, wider and almost verticle tube compared with the left main bronchus. The left bronchus is longer and narrower and extends out at a much sharper angle. This difference is the reason why an endotracheal tube may be positioned in the right main bronchus by mistake and why aspirated material has a tendency to enter the right lung rather than the left one.

The right and left main bronchi further divide into lobar bronchi, and repeated bifurcation continues through segmental bronchi, bronchioles, and several generations distally to terminate in alveoli. The bronchial tree may be thought of as a family tree, where generations are assigned some numerical order. In fact, this is one method of identification widely used, so that the divisions of bronchi can be traced back along the bronchial tree to their place of origin.

Muscle and cartilage maintain the patency of the bronchi. The same type of incomplete cartilaginous rings found in the trachea are present in the main bronchi and the lower lobe bronchi. Cartilage appears to be less complete in the segmental and lingular bronchi in the rest of the lung.

Pseudostratified ciliated epithelium that is rich in mucus-secreting goblet cells lines the bronchi and serves to protect the lungs from dust and bacteria. Below the epithelial layer are two more layers, a basement membrane and the membrane propria.

The membrane propria is composed of loose fibrous tissue that has a rich capillary blood supply. Bands of longitudinal and circular elastic fibers in the membrane help to maintain patency of the segmental bronchi and bronchioles.

Bronchioles. Terminal bronchi divide into bronchioles, which further divide into terminal bronchioles followed by respiratory bronchioles. Dichotomous division continues into terminal respiratory bronchioles and finally into aleveolar ducts, alveolar sacs, and alveoli.

Bronchioles are distinguishable from bronchi because they lack cartilage, and the bronchiolar lining epithelium is a single layer. The terminal bronchioles do not have mucus-secreting goblet cells and cilia, and the epithelium becomes flattened.

Lungs and pleura. The lungs are two conical-shaped structures within the thoracic cavity. Each has a base (the broader part of the cone) and an apex. The right lung is composed of three lobes, the upper, middle, and lower lobes; the left lung has two lobes. All lobes are further divided into segments with a similar distribution in both lungs. To allow space for mediastinal structures and the heart, the medial surface of the lungs is concave. Pulmonary vessels and main bronchi enter each lung at the hilum to form the root of the lung.

During intrauterine life the lungs begin to develop at about 24 days. This occurs somewhat like the growth of a plant, beginning from an offshoot anteriorly of the foregut (which later becomes the esophagus) and proceeding during the first 16 weeks of gestation to form the bronchial structures with tiny end buds. Further growth continues until approximately 24 weeks, when alveolar development begins. At 28 weeks of gestation the alveolar lining structures become finer and more definite.

Maturation continues, and at birth there are 24 million alveoli present in the lungs of an average newborn infant.

The lung is lined by two membranous layers called pleura. Consisting of a thin sheet of collagen and elastic tissue, the parietal pleura lines the entire thoracic cavity. Each lung is encased in the visceral pleura, which is a dense network of collagen and elastic fibers. This tough membrane contributes to stability of lung tissue.

A potential space exists between the parietal and visceral pleura, which separates the membranous layers with a thin film of pleural fluid. This fluid allows the membranes to glide over each other. A negative pressure exists in the intrapleural space, which prevents separation of the lungs from the thorax. Pleural function can be demonstrated easily by placing a piece of glass on top of another piece of glass that has been wetted. The pieces will slide over each other, but it is impossible to pull them apart.

In disease the pleura can become inflamed (pleurisy), or fluid may accumulate in the pleural space resulting in a pleural effusion.

Gas-exchanging lung units. The terminal bronchioles are now considered to be the last purely conducting portion of the bronchial tree where no gas exchange occurs. Structures distal to the terminal bronchioles, which include respiratory bronchioles, alveolar ducts, alveolar sacs, and alveoli, make up gas-exchanging lung units.

Alveolar ducts arise from respiratory bronchioles and are formed by a meshwork of musculoelastic tissue through which alveoli protrude. *Alveolar sacs* are dilated pouches arising from alveolar ducts and are completely lined with alveoli, which results in the grape-cluster effect seen in Fig. 1-1. It is estimated that 14 million alveolar ducts and their sacs are present in the lung.

Alveoli are the most important structures involved in gas exchange. The average adult lung has approximately 300 million. These minute structures are from 1 to 2 mm

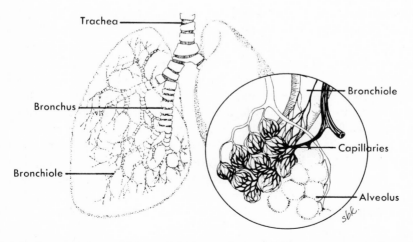

FIG. 1-1. Right lung, cut away to illustrate dichotomous division of the respiratory tract. Insert shows a gas-exchanging unit with terminal bronchiole, dependent alveoli, and alveolar capillary meshwork.

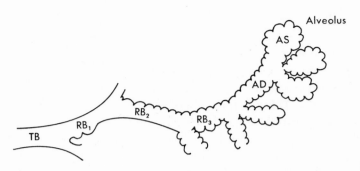

FIG. 1-2. Component parts of the acinus. *TB*, terminal bronchiole; *RB*, respiratory bronchioles; *AD*, alveolar duct; *AS*, alveolar sac. (From Thurlbeck, W. M.: Chronic obstructive lung disease. In Sommers, S. C., editor: Pathology annual 1968, New York, 1968, Appleton-Century-Crofts.)

in diameter when inflated and are often interconnected with neighboring alveoli by stomata, known as alveolar pores. (Alveolar linings and cellular function will be described later in this section.)

An *acinar* gas-exchanging unit is composed of respiratory bronchioles, alveolar ducts, alveolar sacs, and alveoli. Approximately 8,000 alveoli can be found in a single acinus in addition to 400 alveolar ducts and sacs that originate from respiratory bronchioles. Respiratory bronchioles have some alveoli in their walls (hence the name "respiratory" and their presence in the acinar unit) (Fig. 1-2).

Primary and secondary lobule. Dr. William S. Miller in 1937 defined the basic gas-exchanging unit as the *primary lobule*, a definition still preferred by many. The primary lobule consists of an alveolar duct, its dependent alveoli, its vessels, and other structures arising from it (Fig. 1-1). Approximately 400 primary lobules would make up an acinar unit.

A *secondary lobule* is defined as that portion of lung surrounded by connective tissue septa. Each secondary lobule contains between ten and thirty gas-exchanging lung units.

Because of their number and minute size, single gas-exchanging lung units are difficult to see during bronchographic examination with contrast media. Therefore several researchers have been involved in finding a convenient point in bronchiolar anatomy to serve as a cutoff point in terms of a total, functional, visible structure.

Dr. Gamsu and his colleagues at McGill University in Montreal observed a characteristic difference in the appearance of nonrespiratory and respiratory bronchioles, which has led to definite location of an acinar unit. Using special media, they found that respiratory bronchioles had a type of rosette configuration, whereas nonrespiratory bronchioles were small tubular structures.

Alveolar-lining membranes and cellular function. The alveolar surface area is dependent on body size, but in most adults it covers from 70 to 100 square meters and is less than 1 micron thick. It is here where gas exchange between blood and alveoli occurs. Most remarkable is that four types of membranous tissue form this gossamer-thin pathway, known as the *alveolar-capillary membranes.*

Alveolar-capillary membranes have four layers: (1) a continuous lining of squamous epithelium less than 0.5 micron thick, (2) a fine basement membrane made up of elastic fibers and collagen, (3) the basement membrane of the pulmonary capillary, and (4) the endothelial lining of the pulmonary capillaries. A thin layer of interstitial fluid bathes these membranous layers.

Alveolar cells are divided into three main groups: type I, type II, and alveolar macrophages. Type I cells are epithelial cells, which are distinguishable because their cytoplasm lacks affinity for histologic dyes. Type II alveolar epithelial cells are larger cells and appear to occur in the sharper angles amid groups of alveoli. They are highly active metabolically and contain many mitochondria. Type II cells are thought to be the origin of important surface-active material that is responsible for reducing alveolar surface tension. Alveolar macrophages form the third group of cells and are the lungs' garbage disposal units. Their role is important in preventing infection in the lungs (p. 11).

Mast cells. An important group of granular cells known as mast cells is located in the lung, lying just beneath the bronchial epithelium near the smooth muscle and blood vessels. Mast cells are mainly known for their role in releasing histamine in response to an antigen-antibody reaction, such as occurs in asthma. The degranulation process of the mast cells that proceeds as a result of this mechanism has also been found to occur where there is damage to the lungs, for example, as a result of pulmonary embolism or following cardiopulmonary bypass.

Surface tension within the lungs

Surface tension created by molecular forces at the air-liquid interface of the alveolar walls contributes from 50% to 75% of the lungs' elasticity. The existence of alveolar surface tension was first recognized in 1929 by Dr. Karl von Neergaard, at the university clinic in Zurich. He first distended lung tissue with saline, then with air, and measured the pressure required to achieve lung expansion in each case. Dr. von Neergaard found that it took *less* pressure to inflate the fluid-filled lung than was required to inflate the lung distended with air. It was also found that the elastic recoil of the fluid-filled lung was far less than that of the lung distended with air. From this study and the work of several researchers to follow, it was reasoned that something other than elastic tissue must contribute to the lungs' elasticity. These workers concluded that a force—*surface tension*—tended to collapse alveoli and resist alveolar distention.

What is surface tension? Surface tension is a universal phenomenon that exists at a surface of separation between a liquid and a gas (such as at the alveolar surface), between a liquid and a solid, or between two immiscible liquids (such as water and oil).

Tension at a gas-liquid interface results from the activity of molecules forming the top layer of the liquid. Because there are no molecules above them, they tend to be attracted inward and downward, which results in a force pulling toward the center of the liquid. This creates the surface tension. When Dr. von Neergaard filled the lung with a saline solution, he created a liquid-liquid interface, and the phenomenon of surface tension was therefore not demonstrated.

Surface tension can be measured as force per unit length or dynes per centimeter. For alveolar surface area to increase, pressure must be applied. Since each of the 300 million alveoli has a liquid-gas interface, there is little wonder that it takes pressure to overcome the molecular forces at the alveolar surface.

The pressure required to overcome surface tension can be demonstrated by taking a wire ring and dipping it into a soap solution. Pressure by blowing is needed to make a soap bubble. If the pressure is removed before the soap bubble is complete, the soap solution will again fill the wire ring.

Pulmonary surfactant

Pulmonary surfactant is a surface-active material in the alveolar lining fluid. It is a molecular compound called a lipoprotein, which is composed of protein plus the fatty substance lecithin. It is thought to originate from type II alveolar cells. The function of pulmonary surfactant is to reduce alveolar surface tension and thus equalize the pressure within each alveolus during expansion or contraction on inspiration and expiration.

Because of its molecular composition, surfactant acts as fat droplets in water, reducing alveolar surface tension from about 72 dynes/cm (water) to 20 to 25 dynes/cm. It also has the important quality of varying surface tension of the alveoli depending on their size. For example, as an alveolus expands (like the soap bubble), its radius enlarges and the concentration of surface-active molecules is decreased, with a resultant increase in surface tension. As alveolar surface area is reduced, during contraction, surfactant molecules are more concentrated, resulting in a decrease in surface tension. This provides for even distribution of ventilation in larger and smaller alveoli.

Clinically the importance of pulmonary surfactant becomes apparent when it is absent, such as in respiratory distress syndrome of the newborn and hyaline membrane disease. These diseases caused 25,000 infant deaths in 1968 in the United States. But early diagnosis and improved care, particularly during transportation to regional intensive care units, have reduced mortality 50% to 80% in many areas. Such infants characteristically have low concentrations of surface-active material within the lungs. Many other conditions affect concentration of surfactant within the lungs.

Pulmonary mechanics

For gas exchange to occur, air must be brought into contact with the alveolar-capillary membranes. This requires a muscular force to overcome the normal elastic recoil of the lungs and thoracic cage. *Active* contraction of respiratory muscles provides the necessary force to accomplish this during inspiration; expiration is passive.

The diaphragm

The chief muscles of respiration is the diaphragm, which is a dome-shaped sheet of muscle between the thorax and abdomen. The liver is suspended from the right hemidiaphragm. Anteriorly the diaphragm is attached to the ensiform cartilage of the sternum, posteriorly to the lumbar vertebrae, and laterally to the chest wall (lower six ribs). From these attachments the muscle fibers arise in an arch shape and further intertwine with a sheet of connective tissue called the *central tendon*, which then unites with the pericardium. Anatomic structures such as the aorta, esophagus, and inferior vena cava pierce the diaphragm.

Each half of the diaphragm, or hemidiaphragm, has its own innervation—the two phrenic nerves, which arise from the third and fourth cervical nerves. When a phrenic nerve is damaged, paralysis of the affected hemidiaphragm will reduce movement of the respective lung.

Inspiration

During inspiration the chest cavity increases in three directions. The dome of the diaphragm is flattened during contraction with a subsequent increase in the *longitudinal* diameter of the chest. At the same time the external intercostal and scalene muscles increase the chest dimensions *anteroposteriorly* and *laterally* by elevating the anterior portion of the thoracic cage and the ribs. The latter are also rotated outward. The lungs are pulled outward with the chest wall because of their close adherence to the pleura.

Expiration

The process of expiration during normal quiet breathing is passive. The normal elastic recoil of the lungs and chest wall brings the chest to its normal resting position. When expiration is forced or labored during heavy exercise or disease, the internal intercostal muscles draw the ribs and sternum downward. Contraction of the abdominal muscles (rectus, external and internal oblique, and transverse) results in elevation of the diaphragm further into the thoracic cavity, causing a general squeezing of thoracic contents, which actively forces out air.

Pressures within the lungs and thorax

The external pressure exerted on the thorax is atmospheric, which at sea level is 760 mm Hg. When the lungs and thorax are in the resting position with *no* air flow, the *intrapulmonary* (intrapulmonic) pressure is also atmospheric. Intrapulmonary pressure reflects the pressure within the lungs and airways, and this pressure changes with different types of respiration. For air to flow into the lungs, intrapulmonic pressure has to become less than atmospheric (negative) so that a pressure gradient is set up between the atmosphere and the alveoli (Fig. 1-3). *Intrapleural*, or intrathoracic, pressure existing in the pleural space is subatmospheric (−5 mm Hg). This results from the tendency of the highly elastic lungs to recoil from the thoracic cage, creating a vacuum between the visceral and parietal pleurae. If air is introduced into the intrapleural space, the negative "pull" is lost, the lung collapses (pneumothorax), and the thoracic cage expands (Fig. 1-4).

On inspiration it is this elastic recoil between thorax and lungs that must be overcome by muscular effort in order for chest expansion to occur. As the thorax expands

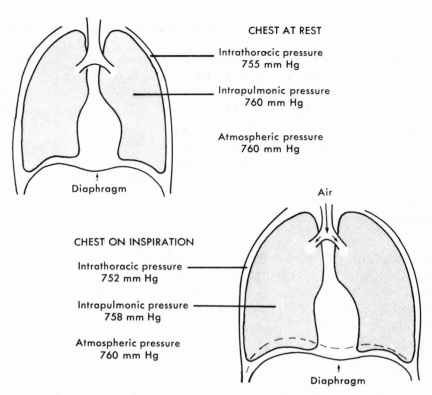

CHEST AT REST

Intrathoracic pressure
755 mm Hg

Intrapulmonic pressure
760 mm Hg

Atmospheric pressure
760 mm Hg

Diaphragm

Air

CHEST ON INSPIRATION

Intrathoracic pressure
752 mm Hg

Intrapulmonic pressure
758 mm Hg

Atmospheric pressure
760 mm Hg

Diaphragm

FIG. 1-3. Pressures within the lungs and thorax at rest and during inspiration.

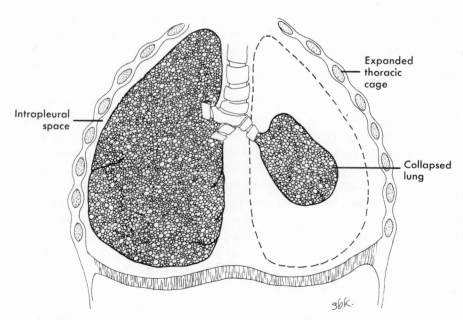

Expanded
thoracic
cage

Intrapleural
space

Collapsed
lung

3bK.

FIG. 1-4. Illustration of pneumothorax. Broken line shows position of normally expanded lung to demonstrate the movement outward of the thoracic cage, which occurs with a pneumothorax.

during inspiration, intrapleural pressure becomes more negative (-8 mm Hg), or subatmospheric, and inflation of alveoli occurs.

Valsalva's maneuver is maximum forced expiration against a closed glottis, which is experienced normally during defecation and parturition where large pressures are required in the abdomen. Initially in a Valsalva maneuver a large breath is taken and held against a closed glottis. As the expiratory force is applied, abdominal muscles actively contract, the diaphragm is elevated into the thorax, and intrapulmonary pressure increases as high as 100 mm Hg above atmospheric pressure. Once breath-holding ceases, the air rushes from the lungs as abdominal and respiratory muscles return the thorax to the resting position.

Control and regulation of breathing

Breathing is controlled and regulated by a fine neural and chemical balance within the body. A single respiratory center is often attributed with the total powers of breathing control, but actually several respiratory centers and receptors are involved.

The *medulla oblongata* of the central nervous system houses inspiratory and expiratory neurons, which form separate respiratory centers. The transmission of all other respiratory center and receptor neural activity is received within the medulla, hence its classification as the primary respiratory center.

Chemosensitive regions are also located in the medulla and are sometimes known as central chemoreceptors. These regions are of vital importance to medullary respiratory control because they are sensitive to levels of carbon dioxide and hydrogen ion concentrations in cerebrospinal fluid.

Peripheral chemoreceptors, known as aortic and carotid bodies, respond to chemical changes in the blood, particularly to decreases in arterial oxygen tension. Hypoxia stimulates the peripheral chemoreceptors, which, in turn, stimulate the respiratory centers to increase ventilation. These chemoreceptors also respond to increases in carbon dioxide levels in arterial blood but are more sensitive to this chemical change in the presence of reduced arterial oxygen tension.

Aortic and carotid baroreceptors also play a role in respiration by their response to increases or decreases in arterial blood pressure. An increase in arterial blood pressure results in a reflex slowing of respirations.

The *pneumotaxic center* in the pons, through its interrelationship with the medulla, gives the rhythmic quality to respiration. It is believed that once the inspiratory center of the medulla is stimulated, neural transmission proceeds to the pneumotaxic center and to inspiratory muscles. Following a momentary pause the pneumotaxic center then stimulates the expiratory center, which inhibits inspiratory neurons and expiration begins.

The *Hering-Breuer reflex* is one of the best known pulmonary reflexes. It aids in the control of respiration because of its effect on inspiratory respiratory depth. As the lung inflates, pulmonary stretch receptors located in the bronchi and bronchioles are thought to activate the inspiratory center either directly or by way of the pons to inhibit further lung expansion. The normal volume of air is thus in part governed by the Hering-Breuer inspiratory reflex.

The *cerebral cortex* provides a center where voluntary control of respiration can occur. This enables us to interrupt normal respiration to speak, laugh, cry, hold our breath, and so on. Breath-holding proves that voluntary control is secondary to spontaneous respiration. As the carbon dioxide buildup triggers the respiratory center via chemoreceptors, spontaneous respiration takes over. (You can probably recall that as a child you tried to see how long you could hold your breath against this powerful spontaneous mechanism.)

Protective mechanisms of the lungs

The protective mechanisms of the lungs are the upper respiratory tract (nose, pharynx, and larynx), ciliary activity, mucus secretion, alveolar macrophages, lymphatics, cough, and airway reflexes. It is indeed amazing that even with the constant inhalation of dust and bacteria, these combined mechanisms are normally able to maintain sterility in the lower respiratory tract.

Air entering the nose carries particulate matter of varying shapes and sizes, which may be deposited in the respiratory tract by impaction, sedimentation, Brownian motion, or turbulent diffusion. The nares (nostrils) contain vibrissae (stiff) hairs that efficiently filter particles larger than 10 μm (micrometers). Once air enters the nasal cavity, it comes into contact with the nasal septum and turbinates. Particles of 10 μm are removed by *impaction*. Most remaining particles of this size are deposited on the nasopharynx because airflow changes direction sharply at this point. Additional impaction occurs in the nasopharynx at the site of the tonsils and adenoids. Should any large particles enter the trachea, these will impact at the carina.

Smaller particles of 5 to 0.2 μm are deposited by *sedimentation* or settling and occur mainly beyond the tenth bronchial division, reaching a peak at about the fifteenth and twenty-third. Sedimentation is possible because of the slow flow of air at these points in the respiratory tract.

Brownian motion is the random movement of microscopic particles suspended in gases or liquids, resulting from the bombardment of the gas molecules surrounding them. Particles of 0.1 μm and smaller are deposited by this method in the respiratory tract.

The size and shape of particulate matter are both important factors when the defense of the lung is concerned. Some extremely large particles (up to 300 μm) such as asbestos fibers may be deposited in the lung periphery. Because of their rodlike shape, asbestos fibers can travel with the inhaled airstream.

Deposition of small particulate matter in the lungs, such as toxic vapors or microorganisms, occurs more readily because they are suspended in the air and therefore more easily inhaled. The danger of such inhaled particles results from their tendency to penetrate the lung more deeply and remain for a prolonged period of time.

Mucus originates from bronchial mucosal glands situated in the membrane propria and to a lesser extent from the goblet cells of the epithelium. Its composition is 95% water, 1% carbohydrate, less than 1% lipid, a small amount of DNA, and 2% glycoproteins (which determine the viscosity of sputum). Normal mucus production during a 24-hour period is approximately 100 ml but can increase to 1,000 ml in disease.

The continuously moving army of sticky hairs provided by ciliary activity is important to the removal of dust particles and bacteria. Each division of the army is in the form of 200 cilia attached to each ciliated epithelial cell. Ciliary movement is wavelike —upward in a single direction toward the trachea. Lying on top of and carried by the cilia is a continuous mucus blanket. The mucus blanket consists of two layers: (1) a lower periciliary fluid layer that bathes the cilia from the surface of the epithelial cell to the apex and (2) an upper gel layer. The gel layer acts as a protective surface that is impermeable to water and prevents to a degree the penetration of toxic substances. Bacteria and dust particles become entrapped in the mucus and are moved upward where they are expectorated or swallowed.

Ciliary activity decreases when mucus becomes thickened or when mucus production increases. Cilia are also affected by pollutants, particularly cigarette smoke, which slow their activity.

Alveolar macrophages are highly efficient in defending the lung through the process of phagocytosis. They are capable of ingesting viable and nonviable material plus endogenously present or exogenously introduced microorganisms. Studies on the efficiency of alveolar macrophages in mice reveal that they ingest bacteria within 5 to 10 minutes of their appearance in the lungs.

Cough protects the lungs by active expectoration of mucus and its entrapped particles. Stimulation of the cough reflex may occur with irritation anywhere in the respiratory tract, and it is a vital defense mechanism when respiratory function is impaired.

Another defense mechanism of the lung is *reflex bronchoconstriction*, which occurs in response to various stimuli such as inhaled irritants (gases, aerosols, or dusts).

Cardiovascular system

Through the pumping action of the heart, blood begins its journey through the vessels of two circulations, the *systemic* circulation and the *pulmonary* circulation. These systems provide for pickup and delivery of oxygen and other nutrients to meet cell requirements and for the removal and excretion of the waste products of metabolism (carbon dioxide and other metabolites).

The heart is a four-chambered muscular organ that is divided into the right atrium and right ventricle and left atrium and left ventricle. Valves separate the atria and the ventricles. The tricuspid valve opens from the right atrium into the right ventricle, and the mitral, or bicuspid, valve opens from the left atrium into the left ventricle.

Venous blood is received into the right atrium from the systemic circulation by way of the inferior and superior venae cavae and is then pumped with the contraction of the right ventricle into the main pulmonary artery and on through the pulmonary circulation. Arterialized blood from the pulmonary circulation is received in the left atrium from the pulmonary veins and is pumped with the strong contraction of the left ventricle into the aorta and then through the systemic circulation.

Pulmonary vasculature. Two circulations supply blood to the lungs. The pulmonary circulation permits gas exchange, and the bronchial circulation meets the metabolic demands of lung tissue. It is interesting to note that the heart and lungs are unique in that they are the only organs of the body to receive the entire cardiac output.

The pulmonary arterial system closely follows the division of the bronchial tree and ends in a dense network of alveolar capillaries that covers a surface area slightly less than the alveolar surface. It should be remembered that the main pulmonary artery arises from the right side of the heart, and therefore pulmonary arteries carry mixed *venous* blood. The pulmonary venous system carries arterial blood and arises from the distal portion of the alveolar capillary bed, alveolar ducts, bronchioles, and pleurae to finally end in the four pulmonary veins, which empty into the left atrium.

The bronchial circulation begins with three or more bronchial arteries, which usually arise from the aorta. It supplies blood to the bronchial wall, the tracheo-bronchial lymph nodes, the midesophagus, and the mediastinal pleura.

Effects of respiration on circulation

With normal inspiration accompanied by the *further* decrease in intrathoracic pressure, blood flow to the right atrium (venous return) is increased, which in turn increases right ventricular filling and output to the pulmonary circulation.

Marked changes in intrathoracic pressure, such as the Valsalva maneuver and mechanical ventilation, have an important effect on venous return. These effects are discussed further in Chapter 10.

BIOLOGY OF RESPIRATION

Once gas exchange has occurred within the lung, oxygen is transported for use at the cellular level in tissue metabolism. Cellular respiration is introduced as a part of this text because of the ever-growing interest in what happens to cells when they become oxygen depleted and the emergency pathways taken within the body in response to oxygen lack. A review of cell structure and tissue metabolism is required to understand certain biologic aspects of respiration.

Typical cell

With the introduction of the electron microscope, significant advances have been made in knowledge of cell structure and function. Fig. 1-5 illustrates the composition of a typical human cell. Three main structures make up the cell—the cell membrane, the cytoplasm, and the nucleus.

Between the cell membrane and the nucleus is the cytoplasm, in which are contained thousands of organelles, comprising mitochondria, lysosomes, and Golgi apparatus.

Mitochondria

Contained within the cytoplasm of all mammalian cells are a number of minute (2 to 3 microns in length) sausagelike bodies called mitochondria. The mitochondrion

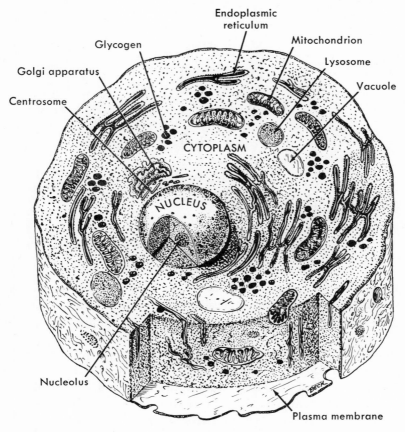

FIG. 1-5. Typical cell. (From Schottelius, B. A., and Schottelius, D. D.: Textbook of physiology, ed. 17, St. Louis, 1973, The C. V. Mosby Co.)

is often referred to as a cell's "powerhouse" because of its high metabolic activity and energy production. Fig. 1-6 illustrates what is seen when a mitochondrion is viewed through an electron microscope. Within the mitochondrion oxygen is consumed and carbon dioxide produced in the process of aerobic metabolism.

Two membranes, composed of lipid molecules and covered with protein, form the mitochondrion; the inner membrane is thrown into folds to form cristae. This unusual structure houses many complex enzyme systems and plays a major role biologically in respiration in the following ways: (1) the oxidation of foodstuffs within the cell, (2) the transfer of electrons from respiratory carrier enzymes (cytochromes), and (3) the production and storage of adenosine triphosphate (ATP), and cell's source of metabolic energy.

Although many foodstuffs are metabolized, only glucose and the end products of its catabolism will be discussed here. Glucose can be metabolized both when no oxygen is present (anaerobic) and in the presence of oxygen (aerobic).

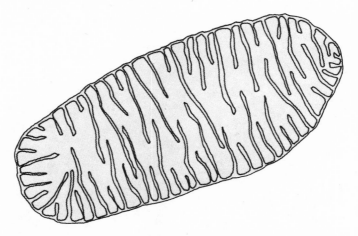

FIG. 1-6. A mitochondrion as seen through an electron microscope.

Anaerobic breakdown of glucose to lactic acid is known as *anaerobic glycolysis.* The last sequence in this series of chemical reactions is the conversion of pyruvic acid to lactic acid. Anaerobic breakdown of glucose occurs within the cytoplasm but outside the mitrochondria.

Glycolysis may be interrupted before the conversion of pyruvic acid to lactic acid, and the pyruvic acid oxidized (aerobic metabolism) to carbon dioxide plus water. This occurs through a series of chemical reactions (the citric acid cycle, or Krebs cycle) and oxidative phosphorylation conducted entirely within the mitochondrion. Briefly, 1 molecule of glucose is broken down by glycolysis to 2 pyruvic acid molecules, which use 6 oxygen molecules to oxidize themselves to 6 carbon dioxide molecules, 6 molecules of water, and 38 molecules of ATP.

As pyruvate is oxidized, electrons are released and transferred to enzyme carrier chains located on the inner mitochondrial wall. The final chain in this series is the respiratory electron-transfer enzymes, the cytochromes. As electrons are transferred along this chain, energy is released and "captured" in the form of ATP.

The respiring mitochondrion thus receives oxygen, which it uses to provide the rich energy bonds of ATP and the waste products of cellular activity: carbon dioxide and water. Clinically the importance of these processes rests with the requirement for oxygen and the functions of the high-energy phosphate bonds of ATP.

ATP has been recognized as one of the most important energy compounds in cellular work. A steady flow of energy is required and is supplied when adenosine *di*phosphate (ADP) combines with phosphate during glycolysis to become adenosine *tri*phosphate (ATP). When oxygen supply to the cell is adequate, 38 molecules of ATP are formed from 1 glucose molecule, but during anaerobic glycolysis only 2 ATP molecules are produced.

In response to oxygen lack, cells revert to the far less efficient emergency pathway of anaerobic glycolysis, which ends in the production of lactic acid. Lactic acid accumulation in the blood is a common occurrence during heavy muscular work, as in exercise and in circulatory failure.

The lung as a metabolic organ

Important progress has been made over the last decade in exploration of metabolic functions of the lung. It is now known that the lung is a highly metabolic organ. Not only does the lung consume large amounts of glucose during respiration but it is also responsible for either the production, conversion, or removal of many vasoactive substances in the pulmonary circulation. Examples are bradykinin, serotonin, heparin, histamine, prostaglandins E and F, and certain polypeptides such as angiotensin I.

Much of the metabolic function of the lung is demonstrated during changes in pulmonary cellular morphology that result from disease or damage. As examples of these conditions arise throughout the text, metabolic factors will be applied.

REFERENCES

Anthony, C. P., and Kolthoff, M. H.: Textbook of anatomy and physiology, ed. 9, St. Louis, 1975, The C. V. Mosby Co.

Bates, D. V., MacKlem, P. T., and Christie, R. V.: Respiratory function in disease, ed. 2, Philadelphia, 1971, W. B. Saunders Co.

Clements, J. A.: Surface tension in the lungs, Sci. Am. **207**:120-130, Dec., 1962

Fraser, R. G., and Pare, P. J. A.: Structure and function of the lung: with emphasis on roentgenology, Organ Physiology Series, Philadelphia, 1971, W. B. Saunders Co.

Negus, V.: The biology of respiration, Baltimore, 1965, The Williams & Wilkins Co.

Newhouse, M., Sanchis, J., and Bienenstock, J.: Lung defense mechanisms, N. Engl. J. Med. **295**:990-999, Oct. 28, 1976; **295**:1045-1052, Nov. 4, 1976.

Said, S. I.: Metabolic activity of the lung and its role in pulmonary disease, Clin. Notes Respir. Dis. **10**:3-9, 1971.

Yoneda, Kokichi: Mucous blanket of rat bronchus, Am. Rev. Respir. Dis. **114**:837-842, 1976.

2 / SCIENTIFIC BASIS OF RESPIRATORY CARE

Persons involved in respiratory care should have an understanding of some basic scientific principles that can be applied to the management of patients. These principles provide a foundation for understanding respiratory physiology and enable the nurse to feel comfortable with many of the concepts presented throughout this text.

GAS LAWS

In the physiologic, or biologic, sense the process of respiration involves the exchange of gases. It is important therefore to have an understanding of the behavior of gases and the laws that best describe that behavior.

Ideal gas law

Under certain conditions of temperature and pressure, gases behave in what is termed an "ideal" way. *Kinetic molecular theory* outlines such behavior and is described as follows.

Gases consist of tiny molecules traveling at high speeds in all directions. This state of high-speed random motion is described as the kinetic energy of the gas, and although gas molecules continuously collide with each other and the walls of their container, no energy is lost. Average kinetic energy of gas molecules is the same for all gases at the same temperature. Gas molecules have no attraction for each other, and the distance between them is large in relationship to their size; therefore the volume of a gas is mainly empty space. A gas volume will completely fill its container and will exert the same pressure at all points of the container.

Scientists have built on the foundation of kinetic molecular theory and have provided simple, workable, mathematical expressions that form the ideal gas law. Many of these are temperature and pressure dependent, so a brief review of these factors will be presented.

Temperature scales

The nurse is generally more familiar with the use of the Fahrenheit and centigrade temperature scales than with the *Kelvin*, or *absolute*, scale. Because absolute temperature is used in the measurement of respiratory gases, a working knowledge of this scale is required.

In 1848 the British physicist William Thomson, Lord Kelvin, developed a thermometric scale with an absolute (perfect) zero. The centigrade scale is divided into 100 equal degrees with the zero at the freezing point of water (32° F) at one end and the boiling point of water (212° F) at the other end (100° C). The Kelvin scale is divided into degrees each equal to the centigrade degree but with the zero at −273° C, and is expressed °C + 273. The boiling point of water is 100° C + 273 = 373° K, and normal body temperature is 37° C + 273 = 310° K. In formulas or equations, T is used for absolute temperature and t for Fahrenheit and centigrade.

Respiratory gases may be measured under various conditions of temperature but are generally reported at the body temperature of the patient. Because of this, accurate monitoring of rectal temperatures (when possible) is important, especially in critical care areas. It becomes vital when patients have arterial blood drawn for analysis. The partial pressure of oxygen in arterial blood has been found to vary as much as 6% with each degree centigrade change in temperature (Chapter 5).

Pressure and the atmosphere

Pressure (P) is defined as *force per unit area*. As gas molecules continuously bombard the walls of their container they exert pressure. Gas pressure is dependent on the number of molecules or moles of the gas present, the volume of the area in which the gas is confined, and the temperature. The pressure exerted by a gas in a tank is measured with a gauge; the pressure exerted by the atmosphere is measured with a mercury-filled barometer.

It was the Evangelista Torricelli, in 1644, who developed the first mercury barometer. He discovered that atmospheric pressure at sea level is great enough to raise a column of mercury 760 mm. Since 1 torr (after Torricelli) is equal to 1 mm Hg, the barometric pressure may be written 760 torr. Because the surface of the earth is at the base of the atmosphere, atmospheric pressure is the pressure exerted by the weight of the air above the earth. Barometric pressure decreases at altitude because the weight of the air is less and therefore the height of the mercury column is less. For example, in Denver, which is a mile above sea level, the barometric pressure is approximately 630 mm Hg; in parts of Himalaya, at an elevation of 19,000 feet above sea level, the barometric pressure is only 344 mm Hg. Such high altitudes reduce the partial pressure of inspired oxygen in the inspired air, thus reducing the alveolar and arterial oxygen levels.

Barometric pressure, abbreviated P_B, may be expressed with other units of measurement, such as pounds per square inch, atmospheres, or inches of mercury:

760 mm Hg = 14.7 lb per sq inch (psi) = 29.9 inches Hg = 1 atmosphere (atm)

Clean atmospheric air is composed of 78.09% nitrogen (N_2), 20.94% oxygen (O_2), 0.93% argon (A_r), 0.03% carbon dioxide (CO_2) and traces of neon, helium, krypton, hydrogen, and xenon.

Moisture in the atmosphere is referred to as *humidity* and is present as a result of the evaporation of water molecules from the earth's surface. This process results in

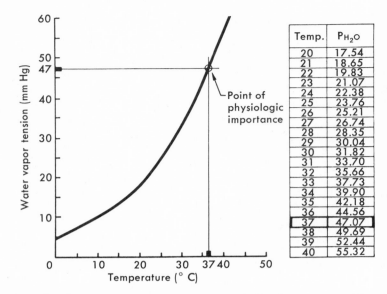

Temp.	P$_{H_2O}$
20	17.54
21	18.65
22	19.83
23	21.07
24	22.38
25	23.76
26	25.21
27	26.74
28	28.35
29	30.04
30	31.82
31	33.70
32	35.66
33	37.73
34	39.90
35	42.18
36	44.56
37	47.07
38	49.69
39	52.44
40	55.32

FIG. 2-1. Relationship of water vapor pressure to temperature. (From Slonim, N. B., and Hamilton, L. M.: Respiratory physiology, ed. 3, St. Louis, 1976, The C. V. Mosby Co.)

water vapor, and the transition from the liquid to the vapor phase results in *water vapor pressure* (P$_{H_2O}$) because of molecular activity. Water vapor pressure is dependent on temperature, and at any given temperature there is a maximum amount of water vapor that a volume of air can hold. When this point is reached, the air is said to be 100% humidified.

The respiratory gases in the airways and alveoli are 100% humidified, and at a temperature of 37° C the water vapor pressure is 47 mm Hg (Fig. 2-1). This is also known as *absolute humidity,* or the actual amount of water vapor pressure present in a given volume of air at a certain temperature. This is important physiologically when the natural processes of humidification are altered either by the administration of dry gases or by bypassing the upper respiratory tract with tracheostomy.

P$_{H_2O}$ obeys Dalton's law of partial pressures (p. 20) and plays an important part in the calculations of *dry gas* measurements obtained from many gas analyzers.

Boyle's law

Robert Boyle (1627-1691) demonstrated that when the pressure on a gas is doubled and the temperature remains constant, the volume of the gas will be reduced by one half. The effect is of crowding gas molecules into half the original area, thus doubling the number of molecules in that area. This results in double bombardment on the walls of the container, hence an increase in pressure. Boyle's law may be stated that at a *constant temperature* (T) the volume of a gas (V) is inversely proportional to the pressure (P), or the product of the volume and pressure is constant if temperature is unchanged. Boyle's law is written:

$$P_1V_1 = P_2V_2$$

Boyle's law can be demonstrated with a plastic syringe with a 1,000 ml volume at a pressure of 1 atm. If the pressure is increased to 2 atm, the volume is reduced by one half to 500 ml. Therefore, if the initial volume is known and the initial and final pressures are known, the new volume can be calculated; or if the initial pressure is known and the initial and final volumes are known, the pressure exerted to bring about change can also be calculated. For example, a mass of oxygen occupies a volume of 2 liters at a pressure of 600 mm Hg. To what pressure must the gas be subjected in order to change the volume to 750 ml? We know that the pressure must be increased because the volume is reduced:

$$P_1 = 600 \text{ mm Hg} \times \frac{2,000 \text{ ml}}{750 \text{ ml}}$$

New pressure = P_2 = 1,600 mm Hg

Charles' law

Jacques Charles (1746-1823) demonstrated the effect of temperature on a volume of gas. He discovered that at a *constant pressure* the volume of a gas is directly proportional to the absolute temperature (T): When gas is heated, the volume is increased; when it is cooled, the volume is decreased. If the absolute temperature of a gas is doubled, the volume is doubled. Charles' law can be written:

$$\frac{V_1}{V_2} = \frac{T_1}{T_2}$$

The first step in applying Charles' law is to convert the recorded temperature to Kelvin. For example, if a volume of oxygen occupies 5 liters at a temperature of 20° C (20° C + 273 = 293° K), what is the new volume if the temperature is increased to 40° C (40° C + 273 = 313° K)? There is an increase in temperature, and so the volume will increase:

$$V_1 = 5.00 \text{ liters} \times \frac{313}{293} = V_2 \ 5.34 \text{ liters}$$

A further examination of Charles' law shows that gases are capable of expansion when heated, thus increasing volume. The French physicist Gay-Lussac in 1802 discovered that all gases expand by the same amount for an increase in temperature of 1° C or contract the same amount for a decrease of 1° C. Interestingly, the volume was found to be approximately $1/273$ of the original volume for each 1° C to which the gas was heated or cooled. This points to the fact that as gas is cooled, molecular activity decreases; at a temperature as low as absolute zero, molecular activity would cease.

Temperature, pressure, and volume relationships can be combined so that changes in different sets of conditions can be calculated:

$$\frac{P_1V_1}{T_1} = \frac{P_2V_2}{T_2}$$

Avogadro's hypothesis and number

The Italian chemist Avogadro (1776-1856) put forward the theory that under certain conditions of temperature and pressure all gases contain an equal number of molecules in a given volume. Because gas molecules are heavier or lighter than each other, depending on the type of gas, the equal number of molecules is calculated on the basis of gram molecular weight, or moles. One mole of any ideal gas contains 6×10^{23}, or *Avogadro's number* of molecules. It was also found that this number of molecules will also occupy the same volume (22.4 liters) at a temperature of $0°$ C and a pressure of 1 atm.

Dalton's law

Dalton's law states that in a mixture of gases each gas exerts a pressure independent of the other gases present and that the total pressure is the arithmetical sum of the partial pressures exerted by each gas:

$$P \text{ total} = P_A + P_B + P_C + P_D + \ldots$$

In other words, each gas in a mixture acts as if it were alone. Under the conditions stated in kinetic molecular theory, gas molecules have no attraction for each other; hence carbon dioxide, oxygen, and nitrogen can all be mixed together in a gas tank.

To apply this law, assume that the gas components of three separate containers, each with different pressures, are to be forced into one container (Fig. 2-2):

$$P_A = O_2 \text{ 140 mm Hg} \qquad P_C = N_2 \text{ 500 mm Hg}$$
$$P_B = CO_2 \text{ 50 mm Hg} \qquad P \text{ total} = 690 \text{ mm Hg}$$

The percentage concentration of each gas by volume is obtained as follows:

$$O_2 \quad \frac{140}{690} \times 100 = \quad 20.30\%$$

$$CO_2 \quad \frac{50}{690} \times 100 = \quad 7.24\%$$

$$N_2 \quad \frac{500}{690} \times 100 = \quad 72.46\%$$
$$\text{Total} = 100\%$$

Dalton's law is also demonstrated by the partial pressure exerted by the different gases in the atmosphere. The total pressure is the atmospheric pressure, but the individual gases all exert their own partial pressure. However, the partial pressure of water vapor must also be considered. The partial pressure (P) of oxygen in the inspired air may be calculated as follows:

$$P_{I_{O_2}} = \frac{\text{Concentration}}{100} \times (P_B - P_{H_2O}) \text{ mm Hg}$$

At sea level:

$$P_{I_{O_2}} = \frac{20.94}{100} \times (760 \text{ mm Hg} - 47 \text{ mm Hg}) = 150 \text{ mm Hg*}$$

(You will recall that at $37°$ C the water vapor pressure is 47 mm Hg.)

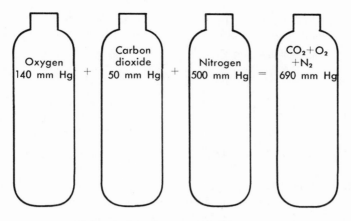

FIG. 2-2. Demonstration of Dalton's law.

At altitude the concentrations of gases in the atmosphere remain constant, but the partial pressures are reduced because the total pressure is reduced.

In respiratory care the partial pressures of gases are spoken of as P_{O_2}, P_{CO_2}, etc., but it is important to adopt the good habit of using correct terminology, so that the person reading the nurse's notes understands where the sample of gas was measured. For example, is it alveolar gas or a gas in the arterial blood or an inspired gas? The partial pressure of the inspired oxygen is written $P_{I_{O_2}}$, and the partial pressure of oxygen in arterial blood is written $P_{a_{O_2}}$. (See Appendix A for the correct terminology.)

Conditions under which gases are measured

When measuring volumes of air moved by a patient's lungs, the nurse applies all the preceding laws for dry gases plus water vapor pressures because gases in the lungs are fully saturated.

STPD. *Standard temperature and pressure, dry* are known as "dry gas" conditions. The temperature is 0° C, the pressure is 760 mm Hg, and no water vapor is present.

BTPS. *Body temperature, ambient pressure saturated* with water vapor are the normal physiologic conditions. The temperature is usually 37° C and water vapor pressure is 47 mm Hg.

ATPS. *Ambient temperature, ambient pressure saturated* with water vapor are the conditions of the room where the gases are measured (generally the laboratory or the patient's room). These must be converted to BTPS, the original conditions:

$$\text{BTPS} = \text{Observed volume (ATPS)} \times \frac{273 + 37°}{273 + t} \times \frac{760 - P_{H_2O_t}}{760 - 47}$$

---

*Actually 20.94% of 760 − 47 = 149.3 mm Hg, but 150 mm Hg is generally acceptable.

If a volume of 5 liters of gas is collected from a patient and the room temperature is 24° C, the P_{H_2O} at that temperature is 22.4 mm Hg (Fig. 2-1), and the ambient pressure is 760 mm Hg, what is the volume BTPS?

$$5.00 \text{ liters (ATPS)} \times \frac{273 + 37°}{273 + 24°} \times \frac{760 - 22.4}{760 - 47}$$

$$5.00 \text{ liters (ATPS)} \times \frac{310}{297} \times \frac{737.6}{713} = 5.39 \text{ liters BTPS}$$

When changing from ATPS to BTPS, the increase in temperature results in an increase in volume (a demonstration of Charles' law). The same occurs when converting STPD to ATPS or BTPS.

Many gas analyzers, such as infrared carbon dioxide analyzers used in the measurement of end tidal carbon dioxide levels, give results in percent of dry gas. The results must then be corrected for the amount of water vapor saturation in the respiratory tract. If a patient breathes into a carbon dioxide analyzer and his end tidal CO_2 is 5.6% at a barometric pressure of 760 mm Hg, the partial pressure is calculated as described for the $P_{I_{O_2}}$ in air:

$$Pa_{CO_2} = \frac{5.6}{100} \times (760 - 47) = 40 \text{ mm Hg}$$

Ideal gas law equation

At this point the work of Boyle, Charles, Gay-Lussac, Avogadro, and Kelvin can be brought together in an equation stating the behavior of ideal gases:

$$PV = nRT$$

Where P is pressure, V is volume, T is absolute temperature, n is the number of molecules in the gas (Avogadro's number), and R is the universal gas constant. This constant is a number that can be expressed in units such as British joules or liters and atmospheres. The value of R will vary with the units used.

When the pressure is in atmospheres, the volume is in liters, the temperature is absolute, and n is equal to 1 mole of gas, R is expressed:

$$R = \frac{1 \text{ mole} \times 22.4 \text{ liters}}{1 \text{ atm} \times 0° C + 273} = 0.821 \text{ liters/atm/mole/° C}$$

The ideal gas law equation is used for the calculation of the number of grams and moles in a gas-occupying volume and is presented here as a united statement of kinetic molecular theory and ideal gases.

Henry's law

Henry's law deals with dissolved gases, or gases in physical solution. In respiratory gas exchange gases are dissolved or chemically combined with the contents of the liquid. Henry's law states that if a condition of equilibrium exists, the solubility of a gas in a liquid is directly proportional to the pressure of the gas above the liquid. In water, plasma, or whole blood, when there is no chemical combination, oxygen, carbon dioxide, and nitrogen are carried in physical solution.

Nitrogen is carried entirely in physical solution, whereas oxygen and carbon dioxide also enter into chemical combination within the red cell.

The law of partial pressures of gases in liquids plays a role in establishing the state of equilibrium applied to Henry's law. Like the partial pressures of gases in the gas phase, each gas exerts its own partial pressure in the liquid phase. When gas molecules are in solution, for example in blood plasma, there is constant activity of molecules passing through the liquid into the gas phase and vice versa. This is particularly evident at the alveolar–blood gas surface, where the partial pressure of the gas leaving the liquid reaches the same partial pressure as the gas entering the liquid; thus a state of equilibrium exists. Although alveolar oxygen reaching the blood is at a higher concentration than the oxygen in mixed venous blood, a point of equilibrium is almost reached by the time the blood leaves the pulmonary capillary. However, other pressure factors and the process of diffusion are also involved.

Henry's law and the law of partial pressures in liquids can often be demonstrated at the bedside. A further discussion of this will be taken up in Chapter 5.

Diffusion

Another property of gases important to respiratory physiology is their ability to *diffuse,* which is the process by which gases spread out and move from one place to another. Kinetic molecular theory states that gases move in all directions. Diffusion can therefore take place up or down or across because of this random movement. It is also as a result of diffusion that a gas will completely fill a container and why an odor will spread throughout a room.

In the body, diffusion of oxygen and carbon dioxide occurs across the alveolar capillary membranes and during oxidative metabolism within the cell. This diffusion is *passive diffusion* down a *concentration gradient* from a higher concentration of gas to a lower concentration.

Diffusion from a gas phase to a liquid phase is affected by the solubility of a gas in a liquid, and Henry's law can be applied (Chapter 5).

Density and viscosity

Two other characteristics of gases are density and viscosity. These affect the flow of gases and liquids within a system. Density of a gas (d) is expressed by weight in grams per liter:

$$d = \frac{Gram}{Liter}$$

The heavier a gas is the more dense it is. For example, the gram molecular weight of carbon dioxide is 44 Gm, and it has a density of 1.96 Gm/liter; oxygen has a gram molecular weight of 32 Gm and a density of 1.43 Gm/liter.

Viscosity is defined as the degree to which a fluid or a gas resists flow under applied force. The cause of viscosity is the way in which gas molecules move during flow and the friction set up as a result of such movement. When flow is *laminar,* or *streamlined,* gas molecules travel in layers in parallel lines; and similar to lanes filled with traffic, some molecules cross over into faster moving layers or lanes, which slows the movement of the molecules in these faster layers.

Viscosity and density both contribute to resistance, and increased pressure is needed to overcome increased resistance in order for the flow of gases and liquids to continue.

Ohm's law

Ohm (1787-1854) explained the behavior of electrical current in terms of the flow of the current through a circuit and the electromotive forces required to overcome the resistance to flow. In the same way the flow of fluid through a tube varies directly with the push behind it and inversely with the resistance offered to it. A modification of Ohm's law is used to describe vascular resistance and airways resistance (Chapter 4).

Poiseuille's law

French physician Jean Poiseuille (1799-1869) contributed much to physiology when he put together the factors that determine the flow of liquids through tubes. These factors become important to nurses because they deal with circulating liquids through vessels and the flow of gases in the airways. Respiratory gases behave much the same way as a liquid at low rates of flow. Poiseuille's law is written:

$$V \text{ (flow)} = \frac{\Delta P r^4}{\pi/8 L n}$$

Where P is the pressure difference between the end of the tube where flow begins and the other end (or $P_1 - P_2$), r^4 is the radius of the tube to the fourth power, L is the length of the tube, n is the viscosity coefficient measured in poises (after Poiseuille), and $\pi/8$ is a constant. The volume (V) flowing through the tube is dependent on all these factors.

A linear relationship exists between flow and the length of the tube; if a length of tubing is doubled, flow will be reduced by one half if the pressure difference in the tubing is constant.

A most important component is the radius of the tubing. The larger the radius of the tubing, the greater the flow; the narrower the radius of the tube the harder it is for flow to take place. If a piece of tubing on a system that had a radius of 6 cm were replaced with tubing of 3 cm radius, the flow would be reduced 16 fold ($2 \times 2 \times 2 \times 2$). Radius is a significant consideration in the asthmatic, for example, because the diameter of the airways is greatly reduced and greater pressures are required to force air through the airways.

When a volume of gas or fluid is to be moved from one part of a system to another, not only the length and radius of the tubing are important but also the viscosity and the type of flow. Flow may be either *laminar* or *turbulent.* Laminar flow is smooth and occurs in straight tubes of relatively the same diameter. Flow may become turbulent when the rate of flow is increased. Turbulent flow is, as the name implies, stormy with the formation of eddy currents. It occurs in irregular tubes, at high rates of flow, and when there are obstructions along the tubes. The irregularity of the bronchial tree causes turbulent flow, particularly in the small bronchi and bronchioles. Gases with high density also increase turbulence.

Large increases in pressure are required to overcome turbulent flow, which occurs in many disease conditions of the chest. This is a factor in the mechanics of breathing and mechanical ventilation.

REFERENCE

Hein, M.: Foundations of college chemistry, Belmont, Calif., 1967, Dickensen Publishing Co., Inc.

3 / PULMONARY FUNCTION

The pulmonary function laboratory plays a major role in the evaluation of lung function in health and disease. Pulmonary function testing requires the full cooperation of the patient, and the nurse is often in the best position to evaluate a patient's ability to follow instructions and to ascertain whether he is strong enough to carry out the study. The nurse is also in the best position to help to prepare the patient for the procedure.

Lung volumes and their subdivisions are simple to understand. However, their application once they are measured is important to total patient management.

This chapter is designed to give the nurse a basic knowledge of a pulmonary function laboratory, the tests conducted, and the nursing care involved in preparing the patient for such testing.

PULMONARY FUNCTION LABORATORY

Although the vast differences that exist among pulmonary function laboratories are far too many to be considered here, there are certain standards and conditions essential to any laboratory when high-quality pulmonary function testing is to be achieved. Some of these standards and conditions include the area where the tests are performed, the persons conducting the tests, and the director of the pulmonary function laboratory.

The testing area should be as pleasant as possible and is best situated where it can be closed off to any interruptions from human traffic. A sign posted at eye level on the door to the area with the words "Do not enter: Study in progress" may help to prevent persons from barging in during a study.

A quiet, unhurried atmosphere without interruptions provides the best environment for pulmonary function testing. Any noise during a study should be prevented. Bells on telephones can be silenced by turning them off; background conversation should be discouraged. Irritating sounds are a constant distraction to patients and have a marked effect on their patterns of respiration. Many studies are carried out with patients in the *steady state*, which requires breathing to be as relaxed as possible. This state is not easily attained when the testing area is crowded and noisy.

Conducting pulmonary function tests

The manner in which a patient is instructed to perform the breathing exercises during pulmonary function testing is the most important factor in obtaining meaningful data. Many tests of pulmonary function depend on the amount of effort that the patient puts forth. Should the instructions not be clear and concise or not delivered with enough enthusiasm, the results obtained will not be a true measure of what the patient is capable of doing.

Only trained personnel should administer pulmonary function tests. This involves giving patients instructions, running the equipment used during testing, and editing and calculating the data obtained.

The staff of the pulmonary function laboratory sets the stage for good rapport with patients and provides a path of communication with the physician involved in interpreting the test results. The way the patient performed the test, the type and quantity of sputum expectorated during testing, and an accurate, pertinent medical and social history are all important facts that a trained person will observe and convey.

In many facilities the pulmonary function department is a part of a cardiopulmonary laboratory, where cardiac catheterization and other methods of evaluating the cardiopulmonary system are carried out. Technologists working in such an area may be trained in the testing of pulmonary function and the methods used in evaluating cardiac disease.

Director of a pulmonary function laboratory

A pulmonary function laboratory should have a director. The qualifications and background of such a person will, of course, depend on the size and location of the facility. The director may be a physician who has a wide knowledge of pulmonary physiology or may be a clinical pulmonary physiologist.

Whatever the qualifications, the director of a pulmonary function laboratory has the responsibility for seeing that testing of patients is done under the best and most scientific conditions possible. A pulmonary function laboratory director should have complete knowledge of laboratory equipment and should be able to train others in the methods used in the testing of patients.

Interpreting data obtained from pulmonary function testing

A physician specializing in chest diseases and pulmonary physiology should be available to interpret data obtained from pulmonary function testing and to write a full report of the findings. This is similar to what a radiologist does when interpreting and reporting findings on a chest roentgenogram.

The nurse plays a vital role in the pulmonary function team, and therefore it is important for the nurse to know what is measured during pulmonary function tests and how and why such measurements are generally carried out.

LUNG VOLUMES AND THEIR MEASUREMENT

A knowledge of the lung volumes and their measurement is necessary to understand basic respiratory physiology and the ways in which disease and other processes disrupt the physiologic status of the lung and so alter function.

A mass of symbols, abbreviations, and nomenclature is used in pulmonary physiology. These are continuously under review and revision in an attempt to clarify them.

The pulmonary terms and symbols throughout this text were compiled in a 1975 report by the American College of Chest Physicians–American Thoracic Society Joint Committee on Pulmonary Nomenclature (also see Appendix A).

The spirometer

Some of the measurements of lung volumes can be recorded with a *spirometer*, an instrument for measuring the volume of air entering or leaving the lungs. A writing device such as a 2- or 4-channel recorder, x-y plotter, or kymograph is attached to the spirometer and provides a graphic tracing of motion at different speeds automatically. A slow speed (30 or 60 mm/min) facilitates measurement of normal, quiet breathing over several minutes. A fast speed, usually in millimeters per second, provides for easy calculation of measurements that involve a unit of time, such as liters per minute or per second (Fig. 3-1). Many types of spirometers and recording combinations are available. A simple water-filled spirometer with a bellows attachment is shown in Fig. 3-1. The permanent record that is obtained with such instruments is of tremendous value. The tracing alone, without a single calculation, provides an

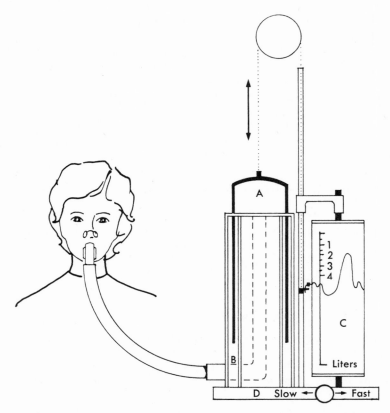

FIG. 3-1. A patient performing pulmonary function test using a spirometer, with bellows, *A*, moving in water-filled area, *B*. The rotating drum, *C*, has a spirographic tracing that can be made at a slow or fast speed, *D*.

abundance of information to the trained eye. Changes in pulmonary function that occur with disease will be discussed in Chapter 6.

Vital capacity and components

Vital capacity (VC) is defined as the volume of gas that can be expelled from the lungs by forceful effort following a maximal inspiration. The vital capacity is an important measurement of lung volume included in spirometry.

The spirograph tracing in Fig. 3-2 shows that the vital capacity can be measured the other way around. The gas is first expelled from the lungs by forceful effort and then followed by a maximal inspiration. This is known as an *inspiratory vital capacity.* Both methods of measurement are acceptable, but inspiratory vital capacity is often preferred when measuring the vital capacity of patients with *air trapping* (Chapter 6).

Hold your nose, relax, and breathe normally. As you come to the end of a breath, just keep blowing out. Get out all the air from your lungs; then take in as deep a breath as you possibly can, completely filling your lungs. Now breathe relaxed. You have just followed the instructions given to patients when measuring their vital capacity.

When these instructions for measurement of vital capacity are followed, it becomes apparent that there are two parts. One part is the maximal volume of gas that can be expired from the *resting expiratory level* (end of a normal breath). This is known as *expiratory reserve volume* (ERV). The second part of the vital capacity is *inspiratory capacity* (IC), defined as the maximal volume of gas that can be inspired from the resting expiratory level. Therefore inspiratory capacity plus expiratory reserve volume equal vital capacity.

In normal persons inspiratory capacity is two thirds of the vital capacity, and expiratory reserve volume is one third. This is demonstrated by the spirograph tracing in Fig. 3-2.

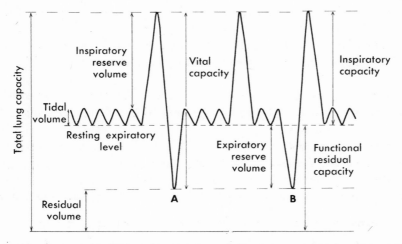

FIG. 3-2. Lung volumes and their subdivisions illustrated by spirograph tracing. *A,* Inspiratory vital capacity; *B,* The more common expiratory vital capacity.

Predicted normal values for vital capacity. Sets of predicted normal values for estimation of the vital capacity have been collected. This was done by testing several thousand subjects of different ages, height, sex, and race. The mean values obtained from such data provide a way to compare a patient's vital capacity with the predicted values. For example, the predicted vital capacity for a male who is 6 feet tall and 45 years of age is 5,000 ml. If such a patient has a volume of only 3,200 ml, there is obviously a marked reduction in his vital capacity.

Many schools of thought exist on what percentage increase or decrease in vital capacity is considered a standard deviation. This question most often arises when a patient's data are borderline. The normal range suggested by some physiologists is ±20% deviation from the predicted normal values.

Tidal volume (VT), or depth of breathing, is defined as the volume of gas inspired or expired during each respiratory cycle—in other words, the normal respiratory pattern (see also Chapter 4). As a component of the vital capacity, tidal volume forms a part of the inspiratory capacity, known as the *inspiratory reserve volume* (IRV), which is the maximal volume of gas that can be inspired from the end inspiratory level (the inspiratory phase of a normal breath).

Accuracy of measurements

When a patient goes to a pulmonary function laboratory for measurement of his lung volumes, it is important that only the volumes of gas within the lungs are measured. There must be no leakage of air from the patient or from the system into which he breathes. A patient breathes into the spirometer with the aid of a mouthpiece designed to fit around the teeth and under the lips to form a seal. This mouthpiece is similar to the type used in scuba diving. A tight-fitting nose clip is also worn to prevent leakage during testing. Leakage can occur if a patient has a hole in his eardrum. The nurse should always notify the laboratory of this condition.

Patients are given a careful explanation of why all this is necessary along with detailed instructions for the measurements to be carried out.

Instructions for measurement of the vital capacity impose no time limit for completion of the exercise. All that is asked is that the patient use maximum effort to obtain the best results.

A patient undergoing pulmonary function testing will always be asked to loosen any tight clothing, such as a belt or undergarment, so that there is nothing to restrict full expansion of the thorax.

Spirometry includes not only measurement of the vital capacity but also measurement of some of the pulmonary mechanics. Here patients are asked to perform breathing tests, at different speeds involving various degrees of force and effort. Pulmonary mechanics will be defined and the measurements explained in Chapter 4.

Residual volume, functional residual capacity, and total lung capacity

Residual volume (RV) is defined as the volume of gas remaining in the lungs at the end of a maximal expiration. Residual volume added to the vital capacity equals the *total lung capacity* (TLC). Since residual volume remains in the lungs even after a person has forced out as much air as possible by voluntary effort, it is not seen on the spirograph tracing and must be measured by indirect methods.

Functional residual capacity (FRC) is defined as the volume of gas remaining in the lungs at the end of a normal expiration. A convenient way to remember functional residual capacity is that one part is engaged in function and the other part is residual. The residual part is residual volume, and the functional part is the expiratory reserve volume. When a physician orders spirometry for a patient, this will not include measurement of total lung capacity because the residual volume will be missing.

Measurement of functional residual capacity and residual volume. Methods of measuring functional residual capacity and residual volume are discussed in detail in many works on pulmonary physiology. It is useful for the nurse to know the names of these methods, but a detailed explanation is not a necessary part of this text. Therefore only a brief description of each method will follow.

FRC and RV are usually measured together because RV + ERV = FRC or FRC − ERV = RV. End expiratory level provides a convenient starting point to begin pulmonary function measurements.

Closed-circuit method. Measurement of FRC (and thus RV) by the closed-circuit method requires the use of a relatively insoluble gas and a closed circuit, such as a spirometer, where a gas mixture can be rebreathed with no contamination from room air. Helium is used in this method and is diluted in a mixture of air and rebreathed by the patient over several minutes. This allows dilution of the initial concentration of gas in the lungs, and so a final concentration is analyzed and the differences calculated. This method is also known as the *helium dilution technique.*

Open-circuit method. The open-circuit technique of measuring FRC requires that a patient inhale a gas from one source and exhale into a collecting system, rather than rebreathing a gas mixture.

The *nitrogen washout technique* is an example of this method. Since about 80% nitrogen is contained in the air, it can be assumed that the lungs contain this amount. Therefore, if a patient inhales 100% oxygen over a period of minutes, all the nitrogen can be washed out of the lungs and the exhaled gas can be analyzed for N_2 content.

The closed-circuit and open-circuit measurements are time consuming, particularly for patients with poorly ventilated areas of lung as in emphysema. Healthy subjects take about 3 minutes to wash out nitrogen from, or dilute helium in, their lungs. A patient with emphysema may take as long as 20 to 30 minutes for every alveolus to be washed out.

Body plethysmography. The body plethysmograph, or body box, is a wooden box shaped to fit the human frame in the sitting position, similar to an individual sauna bath. A transparent dome covers that portion of the box where the head comes through. Once a patient is inside the plethysmograph, the door is closed and the system is completely airtight.

The plethysmograph incorporates the use of Boyle's law of pressure volume relationships (Chapter 2) to measure *thoracic gas volume.* Although values obtained for functional residual capacity with the nitrogen washout or helium dilution techniques are the same in many circumstances, it has been found that the body plethysmograph yields much higher values for patients who have areas of the lung that do not communicate with the outside (for example, where gas is *trapped* in emphysematous bullae or when a tumor occludes a major airway).

Accurate measurements can be obtained rapidly with the plethysmograph. Therefore a patient is not in the box too long, which is important because such a small space soon becomes uncomfortably warm.

Changes in the functional residual capacity and residual volume. Just as the functional residual capacity and residual volume are often measured together, so changes in these volumes in many instances occur together. The most common cause of an increased functional residual capacity is *hyperinflation* of the lungs.

Hyperinflation of the lungs can be caused by changes in lung architecture, particularly at the alveolar level. This occurs with age or pulmonary emphysema. The Greek origin of the word emphysema is *em + physan* (to blow in, inflation), but not all hyperinflation results from the type of destructive changes seen in emphysema. Increase in functional residual capacity from hyperinflation can occur in airways obstruction resulting from asthma and may be seen secondary to thoracic deformity. The significance of these changes will be discussed in Chapter 6.

Changes in total lung capacity. Total lung capacity is the sum of the residual volume and vital capacity or inspiratory capacity plus functional residual capacity. It is clear that an increase in residual volume with a normal vital capacity will bring about an increase in total lung capacity. A decrease in vital capacity with a normal residual volume will decrease the total lung capacity.

CHANGES IN LUNG VOLUMES
Changes in vital capacity in health

Changes in vital capacity in health occur from day to day in the same individual. The variable is usually a small amount, perhaps 200 ml, but it does exist. *Age* causes a reduction in vital capacity because some of the elastic properties of the lung are lost, and the thoracic cage becomes more rigid. A change in *position* from the upright to the supine will bring about a reduction in the vital capacity of 200 to 500 ml. This is caused by a shift in the diaphragm toward the head and a decrease in ventilation at the lung bases.

Pregnancy and *obesity* have a tendency to prevent the descent of the diaphragm, thus reducing the expiratory reserve volume and so the vital capacity.

Changes in vital capacity in disease

Changes in vital capacity occur in many disease states. It is convenient therefore to think in terms of what part of the lung and thorax these disease states affect and to group them accordingly.

Thorax. A restriction to the expansion of the thorax is brought about by structural changes in the thoracic cage in deformities such as kyphoscoliosis and pectus excavatum. Pain and surgical trauma from incisions in the thorax or abdomen, a fractured rib or crush injury of the chest, or anginal pain will all cause a restriction to thoracic expansion and reduction in vital capacity.

Lungs. Pressures and displacement of lung tissue from within the thoracic cavity, such as marked cardiac enlargement, mediastinal tumor, diaphragmatic hernia, or pleural effusion, will prevent full expansion of lung tissue and thus reduce vital capacity.

Conditions occurring within the lungs themselves can bring about a reduction in vital capacity. Examples are pulmonary fibrosis or a collection of secretions resulting from infections such as bronchitis or pneumonia.

Extrathoracic conditions. There are certain conditions that occur outside the thorax that bring about a reduction in vital capacity. Some of these include neurogenic depression by drugs and neuromuscular diseases, such as myasthenia gravis and Guillain-Barré syndrome.

These are just some conditions that can result in reduced vital capacity. It must be remembered that the vital capacity alone will not provide enough information for the total evaluation of lung function. As a single measurement, vital capacity may be considered valuable only when more complete studies have been obtained previously and the degree of reduction or increase in vital capacity provides the necessary follow-up information.

It will be seen later when ventilation, diffusion, and cardiopulmonary circulation are discussed that many more tests are available for the evaluation of cardiopulmonary function.

NURSE'S ROLE ON THE PULMONARY FUNCTION TEAM

The nurse spends the most time with the patient and is in a position of keeping the patient informed and attending to his psychological and physical needs. The nurse helps the patient to have a better understanding of his condition and provides him with an explanation of the procedures he may encounter. The following is a guide to help nurses to fulfill their role on the pulmonary function team.

Preparing patients for pulmonary function testing

The purpose of correct preparation of patients for pulmonary function testing is to ensure that they arrive at the laboratory in the best possible frame of mind and physical condition that their disease will allow. Data obtained under such circumstances can be considered meaningful.

It has been my experience that all too often a patient is rushed from bed in the middle of a meal and whisked into a wheelchair. The first explanation of what is happening occurs when the person transporting the patient says, "Well, off to pulmonary function." The poor patient arrives at the laboratory confused, frightened, and far from being prepared for any test, let alone one for which he should be relaxed.

For the nurse to prevent this situation from occurring, a guideline for the general preparation of patients for pulmonary function testing will be given. In addition, the preparation of patients with special problems will be discussed.

Some of the points taken into consideration when preparing a patient for pulmonary function testing appear to be basic nursing principles. Indeed, some of them are. So many times it is the simple little things in nursing that make a big difference in a patient's progress when recovering from an illness. During the hustle and bustle of hospital life, the little things are often overlooked. Points highlighted here are to serve as a reminder, as well as a guide, to thinking in terms of the *total* patient and his needs.

The patient. What sort of person is he? Are you aware of his needs? Many patients who are scheduled for pulmonary function tests are also hospitalized and going through numerous other procedures. Every time a new face appears at the door to his room, the patient wonders what is going to happen to him next. That old fear of the unknown is always present.

As a result of disease, a patient may have hypoxemia (a decrease in the amount of oxygen in arterial blood). This may give rise to physiologic changes in the brain that further add to a patient's already anxious state.

Not all patients feel the same way, of course. One patient may feel perfectly well and may just be waiting to have a final pulmonary function study done prior to discharge from the hospital. Other patients may be quite ill.

As a nurse, you are the one to make yourself aware of the needs of each patient and to gear your support and preparation of each patient according to those needs.

Timing. Choose the time to prepare the patient for pulmonary function testing with care. The evening before testing is no time for someone to pop into a patient's room and say, "Hi, Mr. Smith. You will be going for some sort of tests for your lungs tomorrow—just wanted to let you know." While that someone is enjoying a pleasant evening out, Mr. Smith is being given all the "information" he needs by the patient in the next bed, Mr. I've-Been-In-Here-Ten-Times-Before.

It is not surprising therefore that the nursing staff learns from the morning report that Mr. Smith got very little sleep last night because he was worried about his lung tests. In this case it would have been better to say nothing than to have had the seeds of fear and doubt planted in the patient's mind.

Ideally, the best time to tell a patient about the procedures is approximately an hour before the scheduled appointment. Explain the types of tests to be done, where the patient will be going, and how long he will be away from his room.

Reasons. Explain why the tests are being done. A patient is entitled to an explanation of why these particular studies have to be done. Patients will often say that they do not have anything wrong with their lungs and, indeed, this may be so. There are many reasons why pulmonary function studies are carried out. This may be a simple baseline study prior to surgery or therapy of some kind (for example, drug therapy, such as steroids, or radiation therapy for a tumor). A patient may not be aware of his diagnosis (for example, if a disease is life threatening), in which case the patient's physician should be asked to help give the patient a satisfactory explanation.

Equipment. What the patient will see? The more elaborate the pulmonary function department, the more strange and overpowering the equipment. A professional can look at these instruments with interest and a detached attitude, but imagine how terrified an elderly lady gasping for air feels as she anticipates having to make every part of a weird contraption move with her little lungs.

Fear is greatly reduced with knowledge. A gentle warning from a kind nurse that these machines are strange looking will alleviate some of the fear and reduce the patient's anxiety. A further explanation that all the patient is expected to do most of the time is to breathe into the equipment so that the air in his lungs can be measured will also make the patient feel more at ease.

Pain. Reassure the patient that this is not a painful study, but warn him that it may be time consuming, depending on what type of test has been ordered. The personnel in the pulmonary function laboratory should be able to provide an estimate of the time that a study will take.

The nose clip, which is worn intermittently throughout the study, may be uncomfortable for the patient. Should an arterial puncture or the placement of an indwelling arterial catheter be required for serial blood gas measurements, explain to the patient that local anesthetic will be used to avoid discomfort during the procedure. Should the patient be allergic to local anesthetic, make absolutely sure that the pulmonary function staff knows this. The tests may be rearranged to minimize the patient's discomfort.

Pace. Never hurry patients. When patients have to leave their rooms for any length of time, they should have a chance to do the things that will make them feel more comfortable. This may be brushing their teeth, going to the bathroom, or being allowed to finish a meal.

Patients should have proper clothing to protect them from drafty hallways during transportation from their rooms to the pulmonary function laboratory.

Anything the nurse can do to prevent the patient from having to hurry should be done. Patients who are already short of breath become more so in any situation in which they are expected to move a great deal faster than usual. It is better to have a patient ready a few minutes early than to have him rushed.

Patients with special problems

Some patients have special problems requiring additional preparation. Such patients may not be able to carry out pulmonary function tests in the normal way, thus making it difficult to obtain truly valid data. The problems encountered most commonly during day-to-day nursing activities are discussed below.

Patients with a tracheostomy. It is not unusual for a physician to want to evaluate the pulmonary status of a patient with a tracheostomy. The physician may want to check the effects of the tracheostomy on lung function, or the patient may have pulmonary disease that necessitated tracheostomy.

The study can be conducted with a *cuffed* tracheostomy tube in situ or with the tracheostomy tube removed and the tracheal stoma sealed as well as is possible. When testing is conducted by way of a tracheostomy tube, the cuff on the tube is inflated to prevent leakage of air around the tube while measurements are being obtained.

The vital capacity is performed in the patient's own time, and for this reason it can be measured easily and accurately via a tracheostomy tube. It is more difficult to obtain an accurate measurement of airflow because leakage of air occurs around even a cuffed tube as air is forced out at speed.

If the tracheal stoma is sealed, the patient can perform the test in the normal way with a mouthpiece and nose clip.

In addition to explaining the procedure to the patient, the nurse should find out from the physician if the study is to be conducted with or without the tube. The pulmonary function staff should be notified that the patient has a tracheostomy so that correct adaptors will be on the equipment when the patient arrives at the laboratory. A suction machine should accompany the patient to the laboratory. Unless the staff in the pulmonary function laboratory or the patient is able to perform correct aseptic suctioning technique, a nurse should be available to assist.

Children. When working with children, a nurse soon knows what a particular child is capable of in terms of ability to follow instructions. Children of the same age may vary considerably in their ability to perform the same task.

Children with asthma or cystic fibrosis may be familiar with the pulmonary function laboratory, since these tests are often used as guidelines in treating and following these diseases. Even the youngest child will have no difficulty in following instructions for the test.

When a child is to have a pulmonary function test, it is helpful if the person who is going to do the testing can meet with the nurse and the child to be studied. They can then work as a team in preparing the child for testing.

Whether a family member should be present with a child during testing is best left to the discretion of the person conducting the study.

Patients with language problems. When patients do not speak English, pulmonary function testing can be carried out easily with the aid of an interpreter. When such patients are prepared, the interpreter should assist with the explanations. It is important also for the nurse to make sure that someone is available to interpret when the patient goes to the pulmonary function laboratory to aid the technician with instructions given to the patient.

Deaf persons can also be studied successfully in the pulmonary function laboratory with the aid of flash cards.

When working with people with language problems, it is very important to notify the laboratory personnel about the patient. It is extremely poor nursing management for a patient to be placed in a position of helplessly trying to explain his dilemma; the situation is also frustrating for those persons trying to help the patient.

PHYSICAL THERAPY, RESPIRATORY THERAPY, AND INTRAVENOUS THERAPY

Physical therapy. When patients are on regular schedules of chest physical therapy, it is an advantage for them to have such treatment before pulmonary function testing. It is important that patients are as free from secretions as possible, and postural drainage and percussion aid in this. However, a patient should not be so exhausted following physical therapy that he is unable to perform the pulmonary function test. Timing of both procedures should be considered.

Respiratory therapy. Patients with chest diseases are often on *intermittent positive pressure breathing* treatments (IPPB), and a treatment may be due just before a patient is to go to the pulmonary function laboratory. Simple IPPB treatment with saline nebulization should be carried out as scheduled so that the patient can eliminate as many secretions as possible. However, IPPB treatment that includes the use of a bronchodilator should not be given before pulmonary function testing. Spirometry is often conducted before and after bronchodilator therapy to evaluate the degree and type of airways obstruction. Therefore it is not advisable for patients to have inhaled bronchodilator therapy at least 4 hours prior to going to the laboratory. Oral bronchodilator agents, depending on whether they are long or short acting, may need to be held up to 24 hours before testing. Certain drugs that are frequently used in conjunction with bronchodilator agents, such as cromolyn sodium or steroids, may be permitted in some instances.

Patients often have their own pocket nebulizers or inhalers. In wanting to do their best at the time of the test, they may take a few puffs to open their lungs before going to the laboratory. This, of course, should be discouraged.

If a patient is receiving continuous oxygen therapy, it should be determined how long he is able to stay off oxygen without becoming distressed or hypoxemic. If possible, the pulmonary function staff should have this information so that they can administer oxygen to the patient as needed.

Intravenous therapy. All intravenous fluids should, of course, be running and of sufficient quantity to last during the time that the patient is away from the ward. If there is medication such as aminophylline in the intravenous infusion, the pulmonary function staff should be informed because the drug affects bronchial dilatation.

There are other special cases and situations that will crop up from time to time. By following the guidelines for general preparation of the patient and by keeping the doors of communication open with the pulmonary function laboratory, nurses will fulfill their role on the pulmonary function team.

FACTORS GOVERNING THE TYPES OF PULMONARY FUNCTION TESTS

The factors governing the types of pulmonary function tests carried out in a given facility are many, but they are generally governed by the law of supply and demand. A fully equipped laboratory is of use only if there are personnel to run it, physicians to take advantage of it, and enough patients to be tested.

Pulmonary function equipment usually varies according to the situation and location. A doctor's office, a clinic, or a small hospital may require only a simple device for measuring vital capacity and some of the pulmonary mechanics. Data obtained from such a device would provide enough information to refer the patient for further, more sophisticated studies or would serve as a tool when serial follow-up measurements are made.

WHY PULMONARY FUNCTION TESTING?

With the increase in noxious atmospheric gases and the high incidence of self-induced pollution from smoking, pulmonary function testing has become an increasingly important part of routine clinical evaluation. Pulmonary function testing now takes its place along with other diagnostic aids, such as chest x-ray examinations and electrocardiograms.

Lung volumes provide much information about pulmonary status. This information is limited, however, because it tells little of the mechanical properties of the lung. Data concerning ventilation and pulmonary mechanics (Chapter 4) can be combined with lung volume data to provide a wealth of information on pulmonary function.

REFERENCES

Comroe, J. H., Jr.: Physiology of respiration, ed. 2, Chicago, 1974, Year Book Medical Publishers, Inc.

Pulmonary terms and symbols: a report of the ACCP-ATS Joint Committee on Pulmonary Nomenclature, Chest **67:**583-593, 1975.

Slonim, N. B., and Hamilton, L. H.: Respiratory physiology, ed. 3, St. Louis, 1976, The C. V. Mosby Co.

West, J. B.: Respiratory physiology: the essentials, Baltimore, 1974, The Williams & Wilkins Co.

4 / VENTILATION, BLOOD FLOW, AND DIFFUSION

The maintenance of alveolar and blood oxygen and carbon dioxide at normal levels requires the integration of ventilation, blood flow, and diffusion. Understanding these processes is essential in caring for patients with respiratory problems, regardless of whether these problems are primary or secondary to respiratory disease. This chapter is not intended, however, to turn the nurse into a pulmonary physiologist but to present physiologic concepts that can be applied to nursing care.

Human beings must breathe in order to live, but air going into the lungs is of no value unless blood is flowing through the pulmonary vasculature to pick up oxygen and give off carbon dioxide. This process of gas exchange is possible only when diffusion occurs across the alveolar-capillary membranes; and once diffusion has occurred, a red cell with hemoglobin must be available to combine chemically with the oxygen provided.

The close link between the heart and lungs cannot be overemphasized. The pumping action of the right ventricle starts the blood on its way for oxygenation, and the left atrium receives the richly oxygenated blood for delivery by way of the systemic circulation to the cell's "powerhouse," the mitochondrion.

VENTILATION

Ventilation is a mechanical process involving the muscular and elastic properties of the lung and thorax that *moves* a volume of air (the tidal volume) into and out from the lungs with inspiration and expiration.

For ventilation to be effective the volume of fresh air brought into the lungs must (1) reach the alveoli for gas exchange to occur, (2) be of sufficient volume to meet metabolic requirements, and (3) have effective distribution throughout the alveoli, with respect to blood flow.

Tidal volume (VT)

During the respiratory cycle only a portion of the tidal volume reaches the alveoli to take part in gas exchange. The remainder is left in the conducting airways and does not take part in gas exchange. This is *ineffective* or *wasted* ventilation. For example, if the tidal volume is 500 ml, only 350 ml would reach the alveoli. The remaining 150 ml would fill the conducting airways, which are said to have a volume of 150 to 180 ml in most adults or are estimated at 1 ml/lb of body weight. This is known as the anatomic dead space (p. 41).

Tidal volume can be measured at the bedside. Mechanical ventilators often have a spirometer bellows attached so that such measurements can be performed routinely. Average normal values for tidal volume vary considerably but usually range from 400 to 600 ml.

Frequency of breathing (f)

The rate, or frequency, of breathing is among the most common of the vital signs and is important in many calculations of respiratory function. However, this measurement alone provides little information on respiratory status.

Minute volume ($\dot{V}_E$)

Minute volume, or minute ventilation, is calculated as tidal volume times frequency of breathing. The symbol for minute volume is $\dot{V}_E$. The V for volume has a dot over it to indicate that time is a factor. The E means that the measurement is made of the expiratory phase of the tidal volume. This is important because expired air is fully saturated with water vapor and the measurement is therefore expressed as milliliters per minute or liters per minute BTPS. For example, if the tidal volume is 500 ml and the breathing frequency is 15 breaths per minute, the minute volume would be 7,500 ml.

Minute volume can be calculated by using a bedside spirometer, or since many mechanical ventilators have flow volume meters attached, the minute volume can be recorded by just the push of a button.

A method used in the pulmonary function laboratory for measurement of $\dot{V}_E$, which is also used at the bedside, is the collection of a patient's expired gas in a large rubber balloon known as a *Douglas bag*. The total volume of gas collected is divided by the number of minutes of collection time to obtain the minute volume. For example, volume of bag = 40 liters ÷ 5 minutes collection time = 8 liters minute volume.

The advantage of collecting gas in this way is that many other measurements can be made at the same time. Expired gas concentrations of oxygen and carbon dioxide can be measured, and since the concentrations of these gases in air are known, the amount of carbon dioxide produced by the patient can be calculated and the amount of oxygen uptake, or oxygen consumption (V_{O_2}), can be determined.

Dead space (V_D)

Dead space (V_D) is a term used frequently in respiratory management, and the nurse should become familiar with its various aspects. The concept of dead space is important in nursing care, particularly when one is managing patients in need of mechanical ventilatory assistance. The volume of the dead space does not take part in gas exchange and is therefore ineffective or wasted ventilation (which may be the best way of remembering the definition of dead space because the term describes the situation).

There are three types of dead space in the respiratory system: (1) anatomic dead space, (2) alveolar dead space, and (3) physiologic dead space. The abbreviation is VD, where V is for volume and D for dead space.

Anatomic dead space. The anatomic dead space consists of the conducting airways from the nose and mouth to the alveoli—in other words, the anatomic tubes that are not involved in gas exchange and where approximately 150 ml of the tidal volume remain as wasted ventilation, or 1 ml/lb of body weight.

Tracheostomy reduces the anatomic dead space by about 50% because of the bypass of the upper respiratory structures.

Alveolar dead space. Once a volume of air reaches the alveoli, three things may happen. Effective ventilation will occur if the air reaches the alveolus and there is sufficient blood to enable gas exchange. However, the volume may reach some alveoli that have no blood supply. In this case ventilation has occurred because the air did reach the alveoli, but it was ineffective because no perfusion took place and therefore no gas exchange occurred. Wasted alveolar ventilation also occurs if the volume of gas that reaches an alveolus is too great for the amount of blood flowing to that alveolus. The latter two conditions contribute to alveolar dead space.

Physiologic dead space. Physiologic dead space is the sum of the anatomic dead space and the alveolar dead space. This is the dead space most commonly determined in respiratory management, since it is a volume of air that is ineffective with regard to gas exchange and alveolar ventilation.

Physiologic dead space is the measurement of choice when assessing the quality of ventilation because the total amount of wasted ventilation is accounted for. Physiologic dead space can also be calculated at the bedside and requires knowledge of the expired and arterial carbon dioxide levels and the tidal volume. In patients with cardiopulmonary disease the physiologic dead space is usually markedly increased (p. 125).

Alveolar ventilation ($\dot{V}A$)

Alveolar ventilation ($\dot{V}A$) is of the greatest physiologic importance because this is the volume of fresh air that takes part in gas exchange. $\dot{V}$ stands for volume per unit of time; A is the abbreviation for alveolar. Alveolar volume is measured in milliliters per minute, which is alveolar ventilation.

Alveolar ventilation depends on depth of breathing (tidal volume), breathing frequency, dead space, and metabolic activity (how much oxygen is consumed and carbon dioxide removed) each minute. It can be expressed as minute ventilation minus dead space ventilation equals alveolar ventilation, or (tidal volume minus dead space) times frequency equals alveolar ventilation. For example:

$$(V_T\ 500\ ml - V_D\ 150\ ml) \times f\ 15 = \dot{V}A\ 5{,}250\ ml/min$$

Alveolar ventilation can be measured at the bedside. This can be done by using the anatomic dead space estimated from body weight. A more accurate method is to use physiologic dead space so that the alveolar and arterial gas measurements are known.

Alveolar and arterial gases must be maintained at optimum levels, and adequate alveolar ventilation is one part of this process. From the preceding formula it is evident that changes in any one of the three parameters will change the alveolar ventilation.

Hypoventilation

Hypoventilation, or alveolar hypoventilation, occurs when an inadequate volume of air enters the alveoli with respect to the metabolic needs of the body. Alveolar hypoventilation is ineffective in maintaining alveolar and arterial gases at normal levels.

If the tidal volume were reduced from 500 to 300 ml, 150 ml would still remain in the anatomic dead space and be wasted ventilation. This would leave only 150 ml for gas exchange with each breath. Because there would be less air reaching the alveoli, alveolar oxygen levels would be reduced and carbon dioxide levels would increase, since ventilation would be inadequate to remove it.

Alveolar hypoventilation *always* results in *hypoxemia* and *hypercapnia* (increased carbon dioxide in the blood) when the patient is breathing room air. Hypoxemia resulting from alveolar hypoventilation can be alleviated by the administration of low-flow oxygen, which will raise the oxygen concentration at the alveolar level to normal. However, the only way for the excess carbon dioxide to be eliminated is by the *restoration of adequate ventilation* so that the carbon dioxide can be blown off.

Hyperventilation

Hyperventilation, or overventilation, occurs when the volume of air reaching the alveoli is greater than that required for body metabolism. For example, an increase in tidal volume from 500 to 800 ml at rest would bring about a significant increase in the supply of air to the alveoli. A decrease in the carbon dioxide level in the blood occurs, but little or no change takes place in the blood oxygen level unless hyperventilation is severe or oxygen is being administered.

Causes of hyperventilation and hypoventilation will be discussed in Chapter 5.

Diagnosis of hyperventilation or hypoventilation

Measurement of arterial blood gas tensions of oxygen and carbon dioxide provides an accurate index of hyperventilation or hypoventilation, and since the pH is usually measured and the plasma bicarbonate calculated during blood gas analysis, the respiratory and metabolic components can be differentiated.

Changes in ventilation are often thought of as conditions that can be diagnosed and labeled by simple observation. It is easy to assume that a patient with a marked increase in breathing frequency is hyperventilating. But breathing frequency indicates little of the quality of ventilation. A patient with alveolar hypoventilation may be breathing at a rate of 50 breaths a minute in a desperate attempt to compensate for a tidal volume of 200 ml. Although observation of the excursions of the chest can give some idea of the depth of breathing, it is still not diagnostic.

Tachypnea means an increased breathing frequency, and it *may* be associated with hyperventilation or hypoventilation. A patient who is breathing at a rate of 50 breaths per minute is considered tachypneic until a diagnosis of hyperventilation or hypoventilation has been made by arterial blood gas analysis.

Distribution of ventilation

Distribution of ventilation throughout the estimated 300 million alveoli existing in the lung is hard to conceptualize. Simple models of ventilation often give the impression that, throughout the whole lung field, each alveolus is a sphere with an equal volume of air supplied to it. Actually, the distribution of ventilation in the normal lung is uneven. In the *upright position* alveolar ventilation decreases in an upward direction from base to apex; this means that alveoli at the base of the lung are overventilated, ventilation approaches normal in the middle of the lung, and little ventilation occurs in the lung apices. This situation is thought to result from gravity because of the weight of the lungs and diaphragm and the changes in intrathoracic and transpulmonary pressures up the lung. When the position is changed from upright to *supine*, distribution of ventilation becomes more even throughout the lung and the diaphragm is shifted headward. During normal exercise, ventilation is increased throughout the lung because of increased tidal volume and hyperinflation of alveoli that are normally closed. If a person stands on his head, the situation is reversed; the lung bases have little ventilation and the lung apices receive the most.

Causes of uneven distribution of ventilation in disease

There are a number of conditions that can affect distribution of ventilation. In disease the conditions that bring about such changes may be of the chest wall, the lungs, the conducting airways, the alveoli, or a combination of these.

Chest wall. Thoracic deformity or trauma to the chest wall from a chest injury or surgical incision affect movement of the chest wall and therefore reduce tidal volume and contribute to uneven ventilation.

Lungs. Loss of distensibility of lung tissue, such as occurs in fibrosis, will cause restriction to movement of the lungs and reduce expansion. Alveolar ventilation will be decreased and distribution will be uneven.

Conducting airways. Obstruction to airflow can occur from partial or total occlusion of an airway caused by cysts, tumors, or secretions, or can result from spasm of the airways such as occurs in asthma. These conditions will result in a decrease in the volume of air reaching the alveoli and cause uneven distribution of ventilation.

Alveoli. Uneven distribution of ventilation can be caused by changes in elasticity (such as occur in emphysema where there is no tonus), thickening of the walls (pulmonary fibrosis), collections of fluid (pulmonary edema), or total collapse (atelectasis).

MECHANICS OF BREATHING

The muscular and elastic properties of the lung discussed in Chapter 1 can now be applied to the mechanics of breathing and ventilation. Mechanics is the branch of physical science that deals with energy and forces and their effect on bodies. This section is devoted to a discussion of the energy and forces used to determine airflow in and out of the lungs. This mechanism is affected by the compliance, or elastic properties, of the lungs and chest wall, the nature of airflow, the resistance to airflow, and pressure changes outside and inside the pulmonary system.

The breathing cycle

The breathing cycle—inspiration followed by expiration—is called *eupnea*. Individuals are usually unaware of the cycle, but it can be interrupted by voluntary effort (for example, by holding a breath or whistling a tune). The involuntary sigh, which occurs about eleven times an hour, plays an important role in hyperinflating the lungs and opening alveoli that are not normally inflated with eupnea.

It has been mentioned previously that the intrathoracic pressure at the resting expiratory level is subatmospheric, or negative (-5 mm Hg), and intrapulmonary pressure is atmospheric. For air to flow into the lungs, the intrapulmonary pressure must become negative. On inspiration the inspiratory muscles increase thoracic expansion and volume and reduce intrathoracic pressure further, which pulls the lungs out because of their close adherence to the pleura. The volume of the lungs is increased, intrapulmonary pressure becomes subatmospheric (-2 to -3 mm Hg), and air flows into the lungs. The alveoli expand and the intrapulmonary pressure increases $+3$ mm Hg to become atmospheric, and flow stops at end inspiration.

At the end of inspiration the forces and energy used to bring about muscular contraction are removed, and the volume of the gas in the lungs is compressed and pushed out. The elastic recoil of the lungs and thorax brings them back to the resting expiratory level.

Compliance

Compliance is the measure of the elastic properties of the lung and thorax. If something is elastic, it should stretch, but a force must be applied. The force once applied may be resisted, and when the force is removed, the elastic that was stretched should recoil.

On inspiration the force applied to bring about stretch is muscular and can be thought of as pressure. The stretch increases volume so that force and stretch can be converted to pressure and volume and measured as the volume change produced by one unit pressure change in liters per centimeter of water.

At the resting expiratory level the lungs and thorax are in opposition, with the lungs pulling inward and away from the thoracic cage. The result is a stretching of the lung tissue and compression of the thorax. This is a balanced position, and the resting lung volume (FRC) reflects this balance. If the residual volume is increased, thus increasing the FRC, the resting expiratory position would be elevated. This situation would occur with loss of elastic tissue in the lung (for example, in pulmonary emphysema), and the result would be a reduction in compliance.

Changes in the elastic properties of the lung will alter compliance and so will changes in the elastic properties of the thorax. This points to the fact that lung compliance and thoracic compliance are separate, but that, because of their balanced relationship, the compliance for each structure is the same and can be expressed as follows:

$$\frac{1}{\text{Thorax}} + \frac{1}{\text{Lungs}} = \frac{1}{\text{Total compliance}}$$

A decrease in compliance or an increased "stiffness" of the lungs and thorax will always necessitate an increase in muscular work to bring about enough pressure to deliver the correct volume for alveolar ventilation. When a ventilator is doing this work for a patient or is assisting him, the prime consideration is effective ventilation— what pressures does this patient need to get an adequate volume of air into his lungs to maintain arterial blood gases at optimum levels?

Patients who have reduction in compliance have a tendency to reduce their tidal volume and increase their breathing frequency to overcome the work of moving large volumes of air.

Pulmonary surfactants and surface tension contribute to the lung's elasticity and therefore compliance. When surfactant is decreased, compliance is also decreased.

Airways resistance

For gas to flow in and out of the lungs, the opposing forces to motion, or resistance, must be overcome. Pressure is required to overcome resistance, and the amount of pressure required varies with the density and viscosity of the gas, the dimensions of the tube (length and radius), and the nature and rate of airflow through the tube (Poiseuille's law, Chapter 2).

Driving pressure, or pressure gradient, is the difference between a high pressure at one point in a system and a lower pressure downhill. On inspiration the driving pressure is the difference between mouth pressure (atmospheric) and alveolar pressure; on expiration it is the difference between alveolar pressure and atmospheric pressure. This pressure is called *transairway pressure*.

Frictional resistance, created by the gas molecules and the walls of the airways through which they flow, is overcome by the driving pressure, which moves the volume of air through them. Resistance can be expressed as an adaptation of Ohm's law:

$$\text{Resistance} = \frac{\text{Driving pressure}}{\text{Rate of flow}}$$

Because the dimensions of tubes and the nature of airflow through them affect resistance, the caliber of the airways and the nature of airflow through them are important. Two types of airflow, laminar and turbulent, were mentioned in Chapter 2. Because of the difference in caliber in the airways, laminar and turbulent flow exist side by side. The term *tracheobronchial flow* has been used to describe this combination in the pulmonary system. Greater pressure is needed to overcome turbulent flow, which generally occurs with rapid breathing and is common when there are obstructions in the airways, such as mucus and other secretions.

Changes in airways resistance

Airways resistance is increased in normal persons with the inhalation of dust particles or cigarette smoke. A marked increase in airways resistance is seen in patients with asthma, which in many instances is reversible with bronchodilator therapy. The increased airways resistance that occurs with pulmonary emphysema is generally not reversible because it is caused by loss of lung elasticity, which leads to collapse of the respiratory bronchioles during expiration. This collapse differs from the generalized reversible spasm of airways as occurs with asthma.

When patients require ventilatory assistance, the nurse should remember that because there is less resistance to airflow, it is much easier to move a volume of air through a short fat tube than a long narrow tube. Laminar flow occurs in straight tubes, whereas turbulent flow exists in irregular tubes. Nurses should think for a moment of the caliber of a nasoendotracheal tube. They will realize that added resistance is often inflicted on the patient during respiratory management. These are considerations that are taken into account when the pressure settings on ventilators are determined.

Measurement of some of the mechanics by spirometry

Spirometry includes not only the measurement of the lung volumes (Chapter 3) but also measurement of some of the mechanics of ventilation. Rather than specific measurements of compliance or resistance, these are overall measurements and are simple, important tests of pulmonary function.

Since mechanics deals with energy and forces and their effect on bodies, the measurement of some of the mechanics of breathing demands that the patient be able to carry out certain breathing tests at different speeds. The patient then has to use energy and force to get air in and out through the airways as fast as possible. A person with normal lungs can blow out from 75% to 80% of his total vital capacity in 1 second and from 90% to 100% in 3 seconds if he blows as hard and as fast as possible.

The measurements of some of the mechanics of breathing include the *forced vital capacity* (FVC). This measurement is performed with a maximally forced expiratory effort, in which the patient forces out his total vital capacity at speed. Other measurements can be obtained from this single maneuver, such as the forced expiratory volume in 1 second (FEV_1); this is the volume of air exhaled during the first second of the FVC.

The fast speed of the recorder facilitates the measurement of the forced vital capacity. For example, if the paper runs at millimeters per second, then the total length of time needed for a patient to expel his vital capacity can be calculated. The percentage of the total volume expelled at 1 and 3 seconds, for example, can also be calculated at the same time.

To obtain the FVC the patient is asked to take in as deep a breath as possible (maximal inspiration) and to hold it for 1 second. (This gives the technician time to change the paper speed from slow to fast.) He is then told to blow out as hard and as fast as he can and to keep blowing out until all air is expelled. Different laboratories

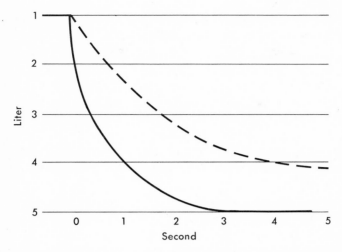

FIG. 4-1. Solid line on the graph illustrates a normal forced expiratory volume. Note that approximately 4 liters of air (80%) are exhaled in the first second and the total volume of 5 liters within 3 seconds. When expiratory airflow is obstructed (broken line), all parameters of volume are reduced, and the length of time it takes for the patient to completely exhale is increased.

may have slightly different ways of measuring this volume, but I have found, and it has been well documented, that it is important to keep the patient blowing out as long as he can.

Some patients with airways obstruction and increased resistance to expiratory airflow (asthma or emphysema) may take from 25 to 30 seconds to expel their vital capacity completely instead of the normal 3 seconds (Fig. 4-1).

Measurement of the forced vital capacity also provides two other values: the forced expiratory flow, measured between the first 200 to 1,200 ml of the vital capacity (FEF200-1200) and the forced expiratory flow between the first 25% to 75% of the vital capacity (FEF25-75%). The terms formerly used for these measurements (and still seen extensively in the literature) are the *maximal expiratory flow rate* (MEFR) and *maximal mid-flow rate* (MMFR).

Patients with obstruction to airflow and increased resistance have marked reduction in both the FEF200-1200 and the FEF25-75%. This is frequently reversible with the use of bronchodilators if the main component of the obstruction is asthmatic in origin.

The *forced inspiratory vital capacity* (FIVC) is measured after a complete exhalation. This is a test at speed so the patient is instructed to take in a breath as fast and as deep as possible, with emphasis on the speed at which the breath is taken in rather than the volume. As a rate of flow it is calculated at liters per minute.

Maximal voluntary ventilation (MVV) is the maximal volume that can be breathed per minute by voluntary effort. The patient is instructed to breathe in and out as deeply and as rapidly as he can for approximately 15 seconds. The MVV is affected by changes in compliance and by changes in airways resistance (because of the increase in turbulence when breathing at high speeds).

Tests for small airway dysfunction

There is mounting evidence that early recognition of obstructive airways disease would be advantageous in providing early therapy that would prevent a more chronic condition. This idea has led researchers to seek methods that will provide such information.

Some newer tests of pulmonary function that are used in early detection of small airways disease are *closing volume* and *maximal expiratory flow-volume curves* and flow-volume loops.

Closing volume. When a normal person takes in a maximal inspiration, all airways are found to be open. As the person exhales and the volume of air in the lungs decreases, the small airways in the periphery of the lungs start to close. The volume or portion of the vital capacity at which small airway closure can be measured is known as the closing volume (CV).

Measurement of closing volume in smokers and nonsmokers has shown that there is an increase in closing volume in smokers; that is, airway closure in the periphery occurs at an earlier point in the vital capacity during exhalation.

Maximal expiratory flow-volume curves. To obtain a maximal expiratory flow-volume curve (MEFV), the maximal expiratory flow ($\dot{V}$ max) is plotted against volume as the patient performs the maneuver of a forced vital capacity. This allows for the direct visualization of airflow at each level of the vital capacity.

Flow-volume loops are graphic representations of airflow plotted against volume during both inspiration and expiration.

BLOOD FLOW

Many of the factors that determine effective ventilation also apply to blood flow ($\dot{Q}$). The volume or quantity of blood must be sufficient and of even distribution with respect to alveolar ventilation.

Blood flow through the pulmonary circulation is dependent on the pump (right ventricle), the distensibility of the distributing and receiving vessels, the integrity of the pulmonary capillary bed, and pressure changes and resistance within the pulmonary system.

The prime function of the pulmonary circulation is to arterialize mixed venous blood. Since oxygen must be brought to the capillary bed and carbon dioxide must be removed for this to occur, alveolar ventilation and blood flow are related functions. This relationship is expressed as $\dot{V}_A/\dot{Q}$. Alveolar ventilation and blood flow are also referred to as ventilation and perfusion and are expressed as a ratio. Before the application of $\dot{V}_A/\dot{Q}$, more must be known of the pulmonary circulation.

The pulmonary circulation is low pressure and low resistance compared with the systemic circulation. The blood pressure in the pulmonary artery is 20/8 mm Hg compared with 120/80 mm Hg in the aorta. Blood flow in the pulmonary circulation begins in the pulmonary artery; passes through pulmonary arterioles, pulmonary capillaries, pulmonary venules, and veins; and ends in the left atrium. This is a one-way flow system with approximately 75% of the pulmonary capillary blood flow occurring during systole and the remainder during diastole. The pumping action of the right ventricle, of course, affects this.

Pressures and resistance in the pulmonary circulation

Just as there are pressures and resistance to airflow through the airways, so there is to blood flow through vessels.

The volume of blood flow is equal to the cardiac output, approximately 5 liters/min at rest. The blood volume of the pulmonary capillary bed at any single moment is from 75 to 100 ml. Because of the distensibility of its vessels, the pulmonary capillary bed is capable of expanding to cope with much larger volumes. For example, during exercise 20 liters/min of blood can be pumped through the pulmonary circulation.

Intravascular pressure is the pressure within the vessels. It may be pulmonary arterial pressure, pulmonary venous pressure, or pulmonary capillary pressure.

Transmural pressure is the difference between the pressures inside and outside compressible vessels. The thin-walled pulmonary capillaries are highly compressible and subject to changes in alveolar pressure because of their close proximity to these structures. They are subject to *intrathoracic pressure*, which also affects the larger vessels (arteries and veins).

Driving pressure, as in the airways, overcomes frictional resistance. The resistance is caused by blood as it forces itself against the walls of vessels during blood flow. In the pulmonary circulation the driving pressure is the pressure difference or gradient between the pulmonary artery mean pressure and the left atrial pressure. For example, if the pulmonary artery mean pressure is 15 mm Hg and the left atrial pressure is 6 mm Hg, the driving pressure is 9 mm Hg.

The resistance that occurs in the pulmonary circulation, known as *pulmonary vascular resistance*, can be thought of as the factors that affect blood flow through the vessels. These factors include the viscosity of the blood, the size of the vessel (length and radius), the changes in pressures in and around the vessels, and the part of the pulmonary circulation in which these changes occur. Pulmonary vascular resistance is calculated on the basis of driving pressure (mm Hg) and blood flow (ml/sec) and is expressed with the same formula used for airways resistance.

$$\text{Resistance} = \frac{\text{Driving pressure}}{\text{Blood flow}}$$

Changes in pressures and resistance in the pulmonary circulation: cause and effect. The pressure in the pulmonary capillaries is estimated at 6 mm Hg and has a critical pressure elevation, which is between 20 and 25 mm Hg. This is important because *acute pulmonary edema* can occur with pressures at this level. When pressure within the pulmonary capillaries is 25 mm Hg, it is higher than the colloid osmotic pressure, and fluid is driven across the capillary membrane into the interstitial space and the alveoli. More will be explained of the details of the mechanisms involved in pulmonary edema in Chapter 10.

In disease conditions, such as left ventricular failure and mitral stenosis, there are increases in pressures in the pulmonary circulation. Left atrial pressure increases because of increased diastolic pressure in the left ventricle. A dam effect is then created, which is relayed back through the pulmonary circulation to the pulmonary artery, with increases in pressure along the way. For the driving pressure to be maintained, the right ventricle must work harder; therefore the pressure is increased, and blood flow is able to continue. This is an important series of events, which may or may not result in pulmonary edema, depending on whether the rise in pulmonary capillary pressure is sudden or gradual.

Pulmonary vascular resistance is dependent on many characteristics of the pulmonary circulation, and an increase in pulmonary vascular resistance is usually a result of the changes in integrity of the pulmonary capillary bed. The capillaries are easily *blocked* by emboli, *compressed* by increased alveolar pressure in obstructive lung disease, *constricted* as a result of alveolar hypoxia, and *destroyed* by disease, as in pulmonary emphysema.

Pulmonary vasoconstriction is produced not only by alveolar hypoxia but also as a result of increased hydrogen ion concentration in the plasma (acidosis). When the acidosis is associated with alveolar hypoventilation and increased arterial carbon dioxide levels, the vasoconstriction is thought to be more pronounced.

All the preceding conditions will result in increased pulmonary vascular resistance, followed by increases in pulmonary vascular pressures (pulmonary hypertension) and increased right ventricular work and strain. Many of the conditions producing an increase in pulmonary vascular resistance are associated with lung disease; right heart disease resulting from this type of pulmonary hypertension is called *cor pulmonale,* pulmonary heart disease.

Measurement of intravascular pressures in the pulmonary circulation

During cardiac catheterization a radiopaque cardiovascular catheter can be positioned in some of the vessels and the pressures measured. The pulmonary venous pressure and left atrial pressure, which are usually the same, may be obtained indirectly by measuring *pulmonary artery wedge pressure.* Since the development in 1970 of the Swan-Ganz balloon-tipped, flow-directed catheter, pulmonary venous and arterial pressure measurements are now conducted routinely at the bedside in the critical care settings of many facilities. Because this is such a widely used monitoring technique, a section is devoted to the subject in Chapter 11.

Distribution of blood flow

In the normal upright lung the distribution of blood flow is uneven and follows much the same pattern up the lung as occurs in the normal distribution of ventilation. There is a gradual decrease in blood flow from lung base to apex with a substantial decrease in blood flow at the top of the lung. As with ventilation, exercise and changes in position from upright to supine bring about more even distribution of blood flow.

It was seen that the pulmonary vasculature is highly susceptible to the changes in pressures in and around it, and these changes affect the distribution of blood flow. In the upright lung the actual weight of the blood in the pulmonary circulation exerts pressure gradients down the lung; this is known as the *hydrostatic pressure.*

The net result of the pressure changes affecting the distribution of blood flow is that the pulmonary capillaries in the apex are almost collapsed because of the effect of alveolar pressure, and blood flow almost ceases. In the middle of the lung, flow increases with an overdistention of the pulmonary capillaries because the pressures within them are greater than the alveolar pressure outside.

Many of the conditions causing pulmonary hypertension and pulmonary vascular resistance also affect blood flow and result in an abnormal, uneven distribution.

DIFFUSION

The concept of diffusion discussed in Chapter 2 can now be applied to the exchange of gases across the alveolar capillary membranes for the arterialization of mixed venous blood. Diffusion is the third component in the maintenance of arterial blood gases at optimum levels.

Passive diffusion occurs in gas transfers because there is a pressure gradient between the gases in the alveoli at one side of the membranes and those in the blood at the other side of the membranes. For oxygen this is the normal Po_2 in the alveoli of 100 mm Hg, which is much higher than the Po_2 of 40 mm Hg in the mixed venous blood.

Diffusion is a rapid process in persons with normal lungs. Oxygen enters the interior of the red blood cell in less than 1 second, and carbon dioxide leaves the plasma in less than half a second. Carbon dioxide diffuses about twenty times faster than oxygen across the alveolar-capillary membranes because it is more soluble than oxygen in the water-containing parts of the membrane (plasma and interstitial fluid).

For the diffusion process to take place, there must be adequate ventilation to maintain the diffusion gradient, adequate blood flow carrying red cells with a normal hemoglobin (so that oxygen can chemically combine with it), and the alveolar-capillary membranes must be permeable to the gas molecules traversing them.

Factors affecting diffusion

Diffusion pathway. Although the diffusion of gases is a rapid process with a diffusion pathway of less than 1 micron, it is rather like an obstacle course through which gas molecules of oxygen and carbon dioxide must pass (Fig. 4-2). For example, the oxygen molecule must first reach the alveolar liquid lining and pass through it, then go through the alveolar membrane, the interstitial fluid, the capillary membrane into the plasma, and then finally through the wall of the red blood cell to combine with hemoglobin. Changes in any of the components of the diffusion pathway will affect the rate at which gas transfers across it.

Certain diseases have been recognized as causing a thickening and stiffening of the alveolar membrane, which in turn causes a reduction in size. Some of these are

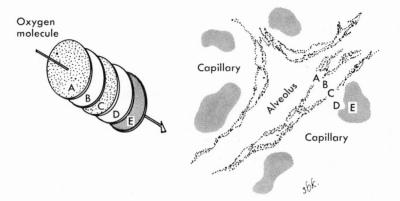

FIG. 4-2. Diffusion pathway shown in stylized form (left) and as seen through an electron microscope (right). An oxygen molecule passes through the alveolar membrane and liquid lining, *A,* the interstitial fluid, *B,* the capillary membrane, *C,* the plasma, *D,* and into the red blood cell, *E.* The whole pathway is less than 1 micron long.

sarcoidosis, asbestosis, and interstitial fibrosis. The rate of gas transfer in these conditions is markedly reduced, resulting in a reduction in arterial oxygen levels (hypoxemia).

Pulmonary edema widens the diffusion pathway because of the increase in interstitial fluid and its outpouring into the alveoli. The result is a reduction in the rate of gas transfer across the alveolar-capillary membranes.

Ventilation and blood flow ($\dot{V}A/\dot{Q}$). Adequate alveolar ventilation and blood flow maintain the diffusion gradient by keeping alveolar and mixed venous blood at optimum levels. Inequality of ventilation and blood flow caused by certain conditions will result in a decrease in the rate of gas transfer. For example, if pulmonary emboli obstruct flow to certain alveoli, no gas transfer will take place in those alveoli. If large numbers of alveoli are destroyed as a result of pulmonary emphysema, no gas transfer will take place in those alveoli.

Severe anemia can result in a reduction in the rate of gas transfer because there is a reduction in hemoglobin available to chemically combine with oxygen.

Patients with ventilation and blood flow disturbances and diffusion defects often present in a similar way, with varying degrees of dyspnea and hypoxemia. The conditions can be difficult to differentiate, a point that continues to be debated by physicians. It is generally agreed that there are both absolute diffusion defects, such as sarcoidosis, and diffusion defects secondary to ventilation and blood flow abnormalities, such as pulmonary emboli and emphysema.

Measurement of diffusion

The rate at which gas transfers across the alveolar-capillary membranes is known as the *diffusing capacity of the lung* (DL) and can be measured in the pulmonary function laboratory.

The single breath technique for measuring the diffusion capacity is carried out as follows: The patient completely exhales. He then inhales as much as he can of a previously measured gas concentration and holds his breath approximately 10 seconds to allow the gas to diffuse. The patient exhales, and the last portion of the total breath is collected in a liter rubber bag and the contents analyzed.

A highly soluble gas is used in the measurement, and the one of choice is carbon monoxide (CO). Oxygen can also be used, but carbon monoxide has an affinity for hemoglobin that is 210 times greater than oxygen. Because carbon monoxide is a highly poisonous gas, a tiny percentage of the gas is used in the procedure.

Once the initial gas concentration is known and the final gas concentration measured, the amount of gas that took place in diffusion, or the rate of gas transfer in milliliters per minute, can be calculated. This is a simple test for ascertaining the degree of diffusion defect and is often used as a monitoring device at 3- or 6-month intervals for patients who have diffusion defects to evaluate the effects of therapy and changes in the diffusing capacity. The term used for this test is DL_{CO}, diffusing capacity of the lung for carbon monoxide.

REFERENCES

Bates, D. V., MacKlem, P. T., and Christie, R. V.: Respiratory function in disease, ed. 2, Philadelphia, 1971, W. B. Saunders Co.

Buist, A. S., Van Fleet, D. L., and Ross, B. B.: A comparison of conventional spirometric tests and the tests of closing volume in an emphysema screening center, Am. Rev. Respir. Dis. **107:**735-743, 1973.

Coates, J. E.: Lung function assessment and application in medicine, ed. 3, Oxford, 1975, Blackwell Scientific Publications, Ltd.

Comroe, J. H., Jr., Forster, R. E., II, Dubois, A. B., Briscoe, W. A., and Carlsen, E.: The lung, ed. 2, Chicago, 1962, Year Book Medical Publishers, Inc.

McCarthy, D. S., Spencer, R., Greene, R., and Millic-Emili, J.: Measurement of "closing volume" as a simple and sensitive test for early detection of small airway disease, Am. J. Med. **52:**747-753, 1972.

Pulmonary terms and symbols: a report of the ACCP-ATS Joint Committee on Pulmonary Nomenclature, Chest **67:**583-593, 1975.

West, J. B.: Ventilation/blood flow and gas exchange, ed. 2, Philadelphia, 1970, F. A. Davis Co.

5 / BLOOD GASES
AND pH WITH CLINICAL
APPLICATION

Maintenance of arterial blood gases at optimum levels is a function of ventilation, blood flow, and diffusion; therefore measurement of arterial blood gases will provide important information on the effectiveness of these processes. Adequate ventilation brings gases into contact with the alveolar-capillary membranes, where diffusion and gas exchange occur. (Oxygen is added to the blood and carbon dioxide removed.) The nurse should also understand how gas exchange occurs at the tissues and the physiologic and chemical factors that influence the behavior of respiratory gases in blood.

WHAT ARE BLOOD GASES?

Blood gases are the partial pressures of oxygen and carbon dioxide in blood. The discussion to follow will mainly apply to levels of these gases in arterial blood. Usually included in the analysis of arterial blood gases are the determination of the hydrogen ion concentration in plasma (pH), the calculation of bicarbonate (HCO_3^-) levels, and the oxygen saturation of blood (So_2).

WHY MUST THE NURSE UNDERSTAND BLOOD GASES?

When the results of a patient's blood gas determination are returned to the ward or critical care area, a nurse is often the first person to see them and should be able to recognize and interpret deviations from normal values. These interpretations should then be applied to the condition of the patient.

Nurse specialists and other personnel involved in critical care should have an understanding of the physiologic processes involved in the transport of oxygen and carbon dioxide in blood and the factors that maintain pH homeostasis. Such knowledge aids in total patient management.

This chapter is designed to provide the physiologic foundations of blood gas transport mechanisms and pH homeostasis, with clinical application and an emphasis on the nurse's role.

OXYGEN TRANSPORT

Thus far you have learned that the human body consumes oxygen (Vo_2) at the rate of 250 ml/min and that oxygen is essential for aerobic metabolism and life processes

54

to continue. You also know that the P_{O_2} in inspired air ($P_{I_{O_2}}$) at sea level is 150 mm Hg, and the P_{O_2} in alveolar gas ($P_{A_{O_2}}$) is 100 mm Hg. Arterial P_{O_2} ($P_{a_{O_2}}$) is normally from 95 to 100 mm Hg but is age dependent.

A difference between inspired and alveolar oxygen exists as a result of the continuous removal of oxygen from inspired air and the continuous addition of CO_2 during respiration.

Oxygen is transported in blood in two ways: (1) in physical solution as dissolved O_2 in the water parts of whole blood, and (2) in chemical combination with hemoglobin.

Dissolved oxygen

The amount of oxygen that is transported as dissolved O_2 is small—only about 0.30 ml/100 ml of blood. The amount of oxygen dissolved is directly dependent on the partial pressure of the gas above the liquid (Henry's law, Chapter 2). For example, if a 100 ml beaker of water is exposed to the partial pressure of alveolar oxygen (100 mm Hg), the amount of O_2 dissolved would be 0.30 ml. If this same 100 ml volume of water is exposed to a 100% O_2 (dry gas) at sea level and 37° C (760 mm Hg − 47 mm Hg), the amount dissolved would be 2.14 ml/100 ml.

If measurements of gases are discussed in milliliters per 100 milliliters of blood (or any liquid), the term volume percent (vol%) is used. The amount of oxygen in arterial blood is approximately 20 vol%, about sixty times as much as in physical solution. If oxygen requirements were to be met solely on the basis of dissolved O_2, a partial pressure of inspired O_2 in excess of 2,000 mm Hg or 3 atm would be required.

Chemical combination and hemoglobin

By far the greatest amount of oxygen uptake and transport is facilitated by *hemoglobin* (Hb), the bright red pigmented protein found in red cells. Iron within the heme portion of hemoglobin combines with molecular oxygen entering the red cells, resulting in oxyhemoglobin production through the reaction:

$$O_2 + Hb \rightleftharpoons HbO_2 \text{ (Oxyhemoglobin)}$$

One gram of hemoglobin is able to combine chemically with 1.34 ml O_2. This is known as the *oxygen capacity* of blood. Oxygen capacity reflects the *maximal* amount of O_2 with which 1 Gm of hemoglobin can combine. In other words, if the P_{O_2} to which the hemoglobin is exposed is raised, no more than 1.34 ml of O_2 could be forced into chemical combination with each gram of hemoglobin.

If a patient has a hemoglobin concentration of 15 Gm in each 100 ml of blood, the amount of oxygen *totally* combined with hemoglobin to form oxyhemoglobin is:

$$15 \times 1.34 = 20.1 \text{ ml/100 ml blood (20.1 vol\%)}$$

Oxygen capacity is mainly dependent on the content and quality of hemoglobin in blood.

Because hemoglobin is so valuable as a carrier of oxygen, physicians are often interested in the *actual* amount of oxygen in combination with hemoglobin as oxyhemoglobin. This is known as *oxygen content* and is dependent on the P_{O_2} to which the available hemoglobin is exposed, and the specific affinity of the hemoglobin for oxygen.

Oxygen saturation and oxygen content

A patient's blood oxygen levels are often given in terms of *saturation*. This reflects the proportions between the actual amount of O_2 combined with hemoglobin (content) to the total amount of O_2 to which the hemoglobin is capable of combining (capacity). The concept is expressed as the percentage saturation of hemoglobin (So_2) and is obtained from the ratio of oxygen content to capacity minus the dissolved O_2:

$$So_2 = 100 \times \frac{\text{Content} - \text{Dissolved } O_2}{\text{Capacity} - \text{Dissolved } O_2}$$

Normally the saturation of arterial blood is 97% and that of venous blood is 75%. Therefore, if the percent saturation is known, the actual amount of O_2 combined with hemoglobin can be calculated. For example, the oxygen capacity of blood is 1.34 ml; if the patient's concentration of hemoglobin is 15 Gm/100 ml and the percent saturation is 97, the amount of O_2 combined with hemoglobin is:

$$15 \times 1.34 \times 0.97 = 19.5 \text{ vol\% content}$$

Oxyhemoglobin dissociation curve

When water is exposed to oxygen at partial pressures of 100 mm Hg and 713 mm Hg, there is a linear relationship (p. 55). In other words, if dissolved O_2 in the water parts of blood were exposed to different partial pressures of O_2 (100, 200, 300 mm Hg,

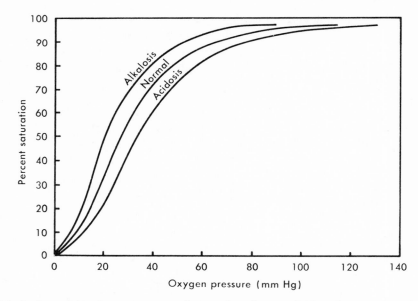

FIG. 5-1. Oxyhemoglobin dissociation curve showing the influence of pH. A decrease in pH (acidosis) shifts the curve to the right; an increase (alkalosis) shifts it to the left.

etc.) and were plotted on a graph, the results would form a straight line. But if whole blood with a normal concentration of hemoglobin is exposed to different partial pressures of O_2 and the percent saturation of hemoglobin is measured, an S-shaped curve is obtained (Fig. 5-1). This is known as the *oxyhemoglobin dissociation curve* and is of great physiologic importance.

When oxygenated, hemoglobin gives the bright red coloring to arterial blood; as it becomes deoxygenated, the color changes to the darker venous blood (desaturated). Hemoglobin at this stage is known as reduced hemoglobin and results from the unloading of O_2 to the tissues.

Significance of the curve. Some of the things to notice about the oxyhemoglobin dissociation curve is that there is an upper flat portion, which is thought of as the arterial portion, and there is the lower, steeper venous portion. The curve is constructed at a temperature of 37° C and at a normal pH of 7.40, which tells us that in some way these factors must influence the curve.

The shape of the curve symbolizes the protective mechanisms in health and disease. When there are fairly large changes in arterial Po_2 (upper portion of graph), there are only small changes in oxygen saturation. For example, if a patient's arterial partial pressure of O_2 drops 30 mm from 100 to 70 mm Hg as a result of pulmonary emboli, oxygen saturation would change only 3% (from the normal 97% to 94%). The hemoglobin can still remain saturated by holding on to its O_2 even when there is a reduction in Po_2. This same phenomenon allows humans to go to higher altitudes where the inspired Po_2 (and thus arterial Po_2) is reduced without any symptoms of tissue hypoxia.

The lower, steeper portion of the oxyhemoglobin dissociation curve offers further protection. As hemoglobin becomes further desaturated from 70% downward, large amounts of O_2 are released for utilization by the tissues with proportionally less change in Po_2.

Influences on the oxyhemoglobin dissociation curve. A normal oxyhemoglobin dissociation curve is constructed under certain conditions and therefore is influenced by changes in these conditions. The result will be an effect on the loading or unloading of oxygen from hemoglobin for changes in arterial Po_2, Pco_2, pH, body temperature, and 2, 3-diphosphoglycerate.

pH and Pa_{CO_2}. A decrease in pH (acidosis) or an increase in arterial Pco_2 will shift the oxyhemoglobin dissociation curve to the right; an increase in pH (alkalosis) or a decrease in arterial Pco_2 will shift the curve to the left. This means that acidosis is accompanied by an increased unloading of oxygen from hemoglobin at a given Po_2 and the reverse for alkalosis.

Changes in pH and Pa_{CO_2} occur through metabolic and respiratory processes. In circulatory failure where respiratory and metabolic acidosis occur concurrently, increased oxygen unloading serves to meet the increased oxygen demand of metabolizing cells.

Temperature. An increase in body temperature affects oxyhemoglobin dissociation in the same way as does acidosis and shifts the curve to the right. A decrease in temperature shifts the curve to the left. Oxygen unloading is decreased, thus increasing the oxygen affinity for hemoglobin (that is, its holding power).

2,3-Diphosphoglycerate (DPG). An organic phosphate known as 2,3-diphosphoglycerate (DPG) plays an important role in the unloading of oxygen from hemoglobin and therefore affects the oxyhemoglobin dissociation curve. Increases in blood levels of DPG result in an increase in oxygen availability, thus shifting the oxyhemoglobin dissociation curve to the right. Levels of DPG are increased in the presence of hypoxia and anemia.

A reduction in the concentration of hemoglobin (anemia) reduces the oxygen-carrying capacity and content of blood. For example, if the hemoglobin were reduced to 8 Gm/100 ml, capacity would be as follows:

$$8 \times 1.34 = 10.7 \text{ vol}\%$$

Content would be:

$$8 \times 1.34 \times 0.97 = 10.4 \text{ vol}\%$$

It is thought that a compensatory rise in DPG occurs in anemia, allowing for more oxygen to be available than would otherwise be in the presence of such a low oxygen content.

Many types of abnormal hemoglobins affect oxyhemoglobin dissociation, and thus transport and delivery. Some of these are fetal hemoglobin (Hb F), Hb Rainer, Hb Kansas, and Hb Seattle.

Carbon monoxide has an affinity for hemoglobin that is 210 times greater than that for oxygen. Oxygen, carbon monoxide, and hemoglobin react to become *carboxyhemoglobin* (HbCO). (Note how the word itself tells something of what occurs when carbon monoxide enters the blood.)

Because of the iron atoms present in hemoglobin, CO and O_2 may be bonded to a hemoglobin molecule at the same time; therefore oxyhemoglobin and carboxyhemoglobin can both be present in blood. This situation is most commonly seen in cigarette smokers, who often have as much as 12% of their hemoglobin bonded to CO. This 12% is ineffective in oxygen transport and delivery.

Normally, blood contains only small amounts of carboxyhemoglobin, and with increases in atmospheric pollution, particularly from exhaust fumes of automobiles, most persons have from 0.1% to 0.3% carboxyhemoglobin present in their blood.

Small concentrations of carbon monoxide, because of its great affinity for hemoglobin, will result in the presence of large percentages of carboxyhemoglobin in blood. For example, inhalation of 0.1% of CO at sea level will result in 50% carboxyhemoglobin in blood, leaving only 50% hemoglobin to carry oxygen as oxyhemoglobin. Exposure to exhaust fumes in a closed area will result in such high levels, as will smoke inhalation.

Arterial oxygen tension

Blood oxygen saturation may be determined when blood gases are analyzed, but the most common, simple, and accurate guide to oxygenation is arterial Po_2, or tension. O_2 saturation is not the best guide to oxygenation because of the many factors upon which So_2 depends and because within the arterial Po_2 range of 60 to 100 mm Hg the changes in oxygen saturation are small.

The nurse is usually interested in the absolute values of arterial Po_2 and the range of Pa_{O_2} obtained for a given oxygen concentration. This points to a further important factor in saturation. Normally, when air is breathed at sea level, the arterial Po_2 is 95 to 100 mm Hg with a saturation of 97%. If 50% oxygen is then breathed, the arterial Po_2 would increase to over 300 mm Hg, but the saturation would have increased to the maximum 100%.

Part of the criteria for defining respiratory failure is a reduction of arterial Po_2 to 60 mm Hg or less. This is considered to be sufficient reduction to be treated at once. However, it must be remembered that many patients never have *normal* blood gas levels but have levels that are adequate for their daily functioning. This is particularly true in patients with chronic lung disease. These patients may have an arterial Po_2 as low as 60 to 65 mm Hg and tolerate it quite well.

Hypoxemia, hypoxia, and anoxia

Hypoxemia is a reduction in arterial Po_2. The term *hypoxia* refers to an inadequate supply of oxygen to the tissues for metabolic needs. The word *anoxia* means "without oxygen" and is often used incorrectly as a substitute for *hypoxia* or *hypoxemia*.

Causes of hypoxemia. There are four main causes of reduced oxygen levels in arterial blood:
1. Ventilation-to-blood flow abnormalities
2. Hypoventilation
3. Shunts
4. Diffusion defects

Ventilation-to-blood flow abnormalities. Abnormalities of the relationships between ventilation and blood flow ($\dot{V}A/\dot{Q}$) constitute the most frequent cause of hypoxemia. When alveolar ventilation is inadequate or unevenly distributed throughout the lungs with respect to blood flow, hypoxemia will result. A reverse situation with the same end result exists when blood flow, either through the pulmonary or systemic circulation, is uneven with respect to ventilation.

Hypoventilation. Whether hypoventilation is primary or secondary to respiratory disease, it is a major cause of hypoxemia. Hypoventilation is defined as a decrease in alveolar ventilation each minute out of proportion to the metabolic needs of the body.

In patients whose lungs are normal, hypoventilation may be considered primary and occurs most commonly after administration of respiratory depressant drugs, such as tranquilizers, morphine, or anesthetic agents. Hypoventilation also occurs frequently in postoperative patients with surgical trauma and pain. These patients limit the movement of the chest wall or diaphragm because of pain, which results in hypoventilation and hypoxemia.

Neuromuscular disorders such as Guillain-Barré syndrome or myasthenia gravis result in severe primary hypoventilation accompanied by hypoxemia. These diseases affect the respiratory muscles and interfere in neural conduction. Patients with these conditions almost always require ventilatory assistance.

Hypoventilation *secondary* to respiratory disease may be caused either by *obstructive* or *restrictive* diseases of the lung (Chapter 6). In obstructive diseases hypoventilation may result from either destruction of alveolar architecture, as in emphysema, or from changes in the caliber of the airways, as in asthma. In restrictive diseases there is limitation to the movement of thorax or lung tissue due to increased "stiffness" (reduced compliance) of the lung or thorax. Pulmonary fibrosis or a chest wall deformity such as kyphoscoliosis will cause this condition and result in hypoventilation.

Shunts. A shunt is classified as either *anatomic* or *physiologic* and always results in the mixing of venous and arterial blood. Therefore there is a reduction in arterial Po_2.

An anatomic shunt is often seen in congenital cardiac abnormalities where left and right sides of the heart are in communication with each other. Shunting of blood occurs in one direction or the other or is bi-directional, mixing blood from both sides of the heart. When blood is shunted from right to left, as occurs in tetralogy of Fallot, anomalous venous return, or transposition of the great vessels, the result is severe hypoxemia accompanied by varying degrees of cyanosis because of such large amounts of venous-arterial mixing.

A *physiologic* venous-arterial shunt exists when a percentage of venous blood bypasses *ventilated* alveoli, enters the pulmonary veins, and mixes with the arterial blood, thus causing hypoxemia (Chapter 8).

Venous admixture, which is a term often used for shunting blood, can be caused by many abnormal conditions of ventilation and blood flow. The difference between venous admixture and the true venous-to-arterial shunt is that in the latter the blood was never exposed to alveolar oxygen.

Diffusion defects. Abnormalities in the transfer of gas across the alveolar capillary membranes constitute the fourth cause of hypoxemia. Absolute diffusion defects, such as occur in sarcoidosis and pulmonary fibrosis, result in thickening of the alveolar capillary membranes and thus reduce the speed at which oxygen molecules traverse the diffusion pathway.

CARBON DIOXIDE TRANSPORT

Carbon dioxide is formed within the mitochondria of metabolizing cells and is produced (Vco_2) at a rate of 200 ml/min. Because the concentration of CO_2 in atmospheric air is small (0.03%), all the CO_2 present in the body results from the metabolic process.

Carbon dioxide is able to leave cells because of the process of diffusion and is transported in blood for excretion by way of the lungs. The process of CO_2 transport, however, involves more than just diffusion and excretion, and the series of events that make up this remarkable transport mechanism will be described. Although a diffusion gradient exists between metabolizing cells with a high CO_2 and blood in the systemic capillaries with a lower CO_2, the gradient in many instances is as small as 1 to 2

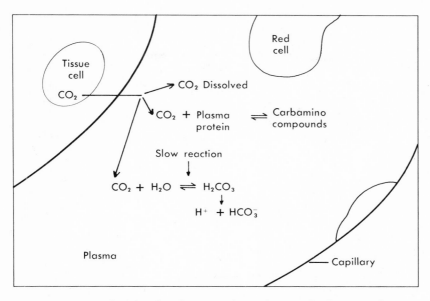

FIG. 5-2. Carbon dioxide transport in plasma. (See text for description.)

mm Hg. Diffusion can take place despite this small gradient because CO_2 is twenty times more soluble than O_2 and therefore will diffuse twenty times faster. Once CO_2 has diffused from cells into the systemic capillaries, it is distributed in *plasma* and *erythrocytes* (red cells) *as physically dissolved CO_2* and in chemical combination as *carbamino compounds* and *bicarbonate ions.*

Carbon dioxide in plasma

Carbon dioxide is transported in plasma as dissolved CO_2 in chemical combination, and as bicarbonate ions. As CO_2 dissolves in plasma, a small amount enters into a slow reaction with water and becomes hydrated to form carbonic acid (H_2CO_3), which then dissociates into hydrogen ions and bicarbonate ions. An almost insignificant amount of CO_2 enters into chemical combination with the amino groups (NH_2) of certain plasma proteins to form carbamino compounds. The largest portion remains as dissolved CO_2 in a ratio of 1,000:1 with the hydrated form. Plasma transports approximately 75% of the CO_2, most of which is in the form of bicarbonate resulting from chemical reactions within the red cell (Fig. 5-2).

Amino acids

At this point a review of the qualities of amino acids will be given because of their importance in buffering systems. Proteins are made up of amino acids, so they are present in plasma and in large amounts in hemoglobin. Amino acids are made up of an amino group (NH_2), which is *basic* in character, and a carboxyl group ($COOH$), which is *acidic* in character. This means that amino acids are *amphoteric*—they can react

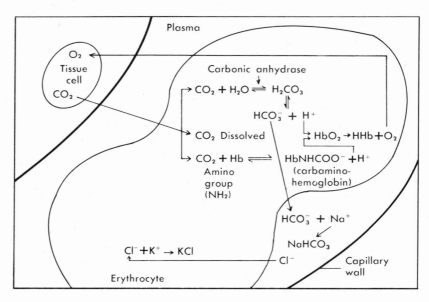

FIG. 5-3. Carbon dioxide transport within the erythrocyte, showing isohydric reaction and chloride shift. (See text for description.)

chemically as either acids or bases. The amphoteric quality means that they can also buffer or neutralize either an acid or a base. These factors are important in understanding the reactions involved in carbon dioxide transport.

Carbon dioxide in the erythrocyte

The greatest number of CO_2 molecules diffuse into erythrocytes for chemical reactions; a small amount remains as dissolved CO_2. Once CO_2 has entered the red cell, it behaves in a similar way to that in plasma with two important differences: (1) a portion combines with *hemoglobin* and (2) the enzyme *carbonic anhydrase* facilitates its transport.

Inside the erythrocyte, CO_2 reacts in three ways: (1) a portion of CO_2 remains in the watery part of the red cell as dissolved CO_2, (2) a portion combines with the amino group (NH_2) of hemoglobin, and (3) a portion combines with water to become H_2CO_3, which further dissociates into hydrogen and bicarbonate ions (Fig. 5-3).

Hemoglobin is a protein that is made up of many amino acids linked in polypeptide chains; an alpha group contains 141 amino acids and a beta group contains 146. As hemoglobin becomes reduced by unloading oxygen to tissues, its amino groups combine with CO_2 to form a carbamino compound called *carbamino hemoglobin*. This is a very rapid reaction, which suggests a bond between the processes of CO_2 loading and O_2 unloading. These processes occur simultaneously both at the tissue capillary level and within the lungs. Carbamino hemoglobin accounts for the unloading of approximately 25% of CO_2 within the lung.

Transport of the greatest portion of CO_2 is facilitated by *carbonic anhydrase,* an enzyme found in large concentrations within erythrocytes. It acts as a catalyst by accelerating the normally slow reaction of $H_2O + CO_2 \rightleftharpoons H_2CO_3$. Since further dissociation takes place into $HCO_3^- + H^+$, the full chemical reaction is written:

$$CO_2 + H_2O \underset{\text{anhydrase}}{\overset{\text{Carbonic}}{\rightleftharpoons}} H_2CO_3 \rightleftharpoons HCO_3^- + H^+$$

The speed at which this reaction occurs is important physiologically because it allows carbon dioxide to be taken up from the tissues in less than 1 second. Excretion of CO_2 from the lungs occurs by the reverse of this reaction in the pulmonary capillaries:

$$HCO_3^- + H^+ \rightleftharpoons H_2CO_3 \underset{\text{anhydrase}}{\overset{\text{Carbonic}}{\rightleftharpoons}} CO_2 + H_2O$$

CO_2 is unloaded for excretion in less than 1 second. In the absence of carbonic anhydrase, this process may take up to 200 seconds.

Isohydric reaction and chloride shift

In the chemical reactions resulting in carbamino compounds and the reaction speeded by carbonic anhydrase, large numbers of hydrogen and bicarbonate ions are formed, which are removed from within the red cell in the following ways.

The hydrogen ions formed are buffered (accepted and neutralized) by portions of the hemoglobin molecules in their different forms. Diffusion of carbon dioxide into capillary blood and the subsequent increase in H^+ is accompanied by a reduction of *some* oxyhemoglobin to form weak acids. These acids are able to buffer H^+, thus forming $HHbO_2$. As $HHbO_2$ gives up more oxygen, it becomes reduced hemoglobin (HHb). The hemoglobin buffering mechanism is so complete that there is little change in the pH; this is known as the *isohydric reaction* (Fig. 5-3).

Bicarbonate ions resulting from carbonic acid dissociation unite with another hemoglobin buffer, potassium hemoglobin (KHb), to form potassium bicarbonate ($KHCO_3$) and reduced hemoglobin. As potassium bicarbonate ionizes, an HCO_3^- gradient is set up between the erythrocytes (red cells) and plasma; bicarbonate ions diffuse *out into plasma* until equilibrium is established between red cell HCO_3^- and plasma HCO_3^-. For electrical neutrality to be maintained within the erythrocyte, the diffusion of HCO_3^- anions into the plasma should be accompanied by diffusion of the same number of anions into the erythrocyte. A phenomenon known as the *chloride shift* allows the passage of a chloride ion from plasma NaCl into the red cell in exchange for an HCO_3^- ion. Once in the red cell, Cl^- combines with K^+ to become KCl, and the HCO_3^- combines with plasma Na to become $NaHCO_3$.

The results of these processes are physically dissolved CO_2, carbonic acid, and sodium bicarbonate, which are all forms of CO_2. Therefore the sum of these equals *total* CO_2 in blood, which in arterial blood is normally 56.3 vol%. This is known as the sum of *combined* CO_2 and *dissolved* CO_2. Combined CO_2 is transported in chemical combination as $NaHCO_3$ and normally equals 53.5 vol%. The difference between total CO_2 and combined CO_2 (2.8 vol%) represents the amount of *carbonic acid* present in plasma related to CO_2 in physical solution, and is known as dissolved CO_2. The partial pressure exerted by CO_2 in these forms is 40 mm Hg in arterial blood and 46 mm Hg in mixed venous blood.

Carbon dioxide transport is dependent on the amount of CO_2 in the blood and the integrity of the transport system. An increase in the amount of CO_2 produced each minute (VCO_2) will result in an increase in H_2CO_3 and $NaHCO_3$. The ratio of sodium bicarbonate to carbonic acid (normally 20:1) provides the foundation for acid-base balance and pH homeostasis.

pH HOMEOSTASIS

Body cells normally function in a slightly alkaline environment (pH 7.40). The stability of this environment depends on normal functioning of the lungs, kidneys, and body buffer systems. Normally the lungs excrete carbonic acid at a rate of 13,000 mEq per day, and the kidneys excrete from 40 to 80 mEq of fixed acids each day.

Acids and bases

An *acid* is a substance that increases hydrogen ion concentration and is a proton donor. The acids present in the human body are of different strengths, which affects the way they behave in solution. For example, a strong acid such as hydrochloric acid (HCl) dissociates completely into free hydrogen ions:

$$\text{(Strong acid) HCL} \longrightarrow H^+ + Cl^-$$

Carbonic acid is a weaker acid because it exists half dissociated and half undissociated, thus donating fewer hydrogen ions:

$$\text{(Weak acid) } H_2CO_3 \rightleftharpoons H^+ + HCO_3^-$$

A *base* is a substance that combines with H^+ and is a proton *acceptor*. A base is known as a substance that liberates hydroxyl ions (OH^-) as it dissociates in solution. The carbamino compounds have this quality.

pH derivation

The number of hydrogen and hydroxyl ions present in a solution determines its acidity or alkalinity. When equal numbers of each are present in water at 24° C, the pH is 7.0, which is known as electrical neutrality. pH is the *negative logarithm of the* H^+ *concentration*. At pH 7.0, H^+ concentration is 1/10,000,000 of a mole per liter, or 10^{-7}; the concentration is the same for OH^-. Because these numbers are so cumbersome to work with, the mathematical scale of acidity or alkalinity is used— the pH scale. The letters pH are used because one of the first papers about hydrogen ion activity, written in French, used the term *puissance hydrogène*, meaning the power of the hydrogen ion.

An *increase* in H^+ will reflect a decrease in pH (acidosis). A *decrease* in H^+ will reflect an increase in pH (alkalosis).

Buffering mechanisms

A buffer is a solution containing a salt of a weak acid or base and is able to prevent or reduce any drastic changes in pH when a stronger acid or base is added to the solution. Buffering systems are made up of buffer pairs. Several buffer systems are present within the body. Three of the most important are (1) the carbonic acid–sodium bicarbonate system, (2) the hemoglobin system, and (3) the phosphate system. Proteins, sodium bicarbonate, phosphates, and potassium bicarbonate contained in these systems are capable of buffering free H^+ and HO^-. Buffering results in neutralization and equilibrium.

In plasma certain *fixed acids* are present, some of which are lactate, inorganic phosphate, sulfate, and ketone bodies. These acids exist normally in small concentrations and are neutralized by HCO_3^- and plasma proteins. Such acids are products of various types of metabolism. Therefore changes in their concentration will result in metabolic acidosis of alkalosis.

Henderson-Hasselbalch equation

The Henderson-Hasselbalch equation is a mathematical expression of the three parameters reflecting acid-base status. (The derivation is given in Appendix B.) The principle of this equation is that the ratio of base to acid, or HCO_3^- to CO_2 (20:1), determines pH. A simplified form of the equation may be written:

$$pH = pK + \log \frac{Base}{Acid} \text{ or } \frac{Kidney}{Lung}$$

pK is the dissociation constant of a buffer system, which for this system is 6.1:

$$pH = 6.1 + \log \frac{HCO_3^- \text{ mEq/liter}}{P_{CO_2} \text{ mm Hg} \times 0.03}$$

To convert P_{CO_2} to the same units as HCO_3^- (either millimoles or milliequivalents), a correction factor of 0.03 is applied. A normal value for HCO_3^- is 24 mEq/liter and a P_{CO_2} is normally 40 mm Hg ($40 \times .03 = 1.2$). Therefore:

$$pH = 6.1 + \log \frac{24}{1.2}$$
$$= 6.1 + \log 20$$
$$= 6.1 + 1.30$$
$$= 7.40$$

At the bedside the nurse would not normally be working with logarithmic tables. However, the Henderson-Hasselbalch equation is the foundation on which many acid-base calculations, nomograms, and graphs are constructed, and it is important for the nurse to understand its application.

Respiratory and renal control of pH

Respiratory control. Adequate alveolar ventilation maintains alveolar and arterial P_{CO_2} at 40 mm Hg and arterial P_{O_2} at 95 to 100 mm Hg. Carbon dioxide is the most important chemical factor in respiratory control of P_{CO_2} and H^+ concentration and their ultimate effect on pH-sensitive respiratory chemoreceptors.

As arterial P_{CO_2} increases (hypercapnia), H^+ concentration increases and pH falls. This results in an increase in the hydrogen ion concentration in cerebrospinal fluid. Respiratory chemoreceptors respond with an immediate increase in respiratory drive, thus increasing alveolar ventilation and removing excess carbon dioxide. An initial decrease in arterial P_{CO_2} causes an increase in pH and reduction of hydrogen ions; respiratory drive is slowed and alveolar ventilation decreases, which restores P_{CO_2} to a higher level.

A rapid increase in arterial P_{CO_2} to 80 mm Hg has a narcotic effect on the central nervous system that results in drowsiness and confusion. If the condition worsens, the result will be unconsciousness and coma. Increases in H^+ concentration by the addition of large amounts of fixed acids have the same effect as increased P_{CO_2}. This is clearly demonstrated with the Kussmaul respirations seen in diabetic ketoacidosis.

Arterial P_{O_2} also regulates the respiratory control of pH by its effects on the chemoreceptors of the carotid and aortic bodies. When oxygen tension is within normal range, there is a regulated low-frequency flow of impulses sent to the respiratory centers within the medulla. A decrease in arterial P_{O_2} increases the flow of impulses, resulting in an increase in ventilation. A *sudden* increase in arterial P_{O_2} results in a decrease in the flow of impulses from the carotid and aortic bodies, thus a decrease in ventilation. The resulting increased arterial P_{CO_2} and the increased H^+ will in turn stimulate respiration so that a normal balance is established. When arterial P_{O_2} falls to 60 mm Hg or below, the hypoxic drive to respiration is the stronger reflex; this becomes important when an increase in carbon dioxide and decreased oxygen tension exist side by side (Chapter 8).

Renal control of pH. The kidneys are able to regulate electrolyte balance and the acidity or alkalinity of the urine. When H^+ concentration in arterial blood is increased (decreased pH), the renal tubules immediately respond by excreting more hydrogen ions and thus a more acid urine. For every H^+ excreted in the urine a basic ion is absorbed, which results in an increase in base and a higher arterial pH. The following stepwise processes accomplish this.

Carbon dioxide diffuses from renal capillaries into renal tubular cells, where it is hydrated through the reaction:

$$CO_2 + H_2O \rightleftharpoons H_2CO_3 \rightleftharpoons HCO_3^- + H^+$$

This reaction is sped by carbonic anhydrase. The hydrogen ions that are formed diffuse into collecting tubules in exchange for sodium ions, which then unite with bicarbonate to become $NaHCO_3$.

When hypercapnia persists, this process will allow full renal compensation for the increase in H^+. In other words, H^+ will continue to be excreted and sodium bicarbonate reabsorbed until arterial pH is normal. Potassium ions are also excreted in the urine, and rapid excretion of hydrogen ions results in less K^+ excretion, hence potassium retention. This is particularly so in respiratory acidosis.

Just as the blood has buffers so does the urine, in forms of phosphate (HPO_4^-) and ammonia (NH_3). Ammonia is formed in the tubular cells from amino acids and gluta-mine and is excreted into tubular urine, where it accepts H^+. The result is ammonium ions (NH_4^+) accompanied by displacement of sodium or some other basic ion, which is then reabsorbed.

Renal compensation to restore pH is a slow process, whereas respiratory com-pensation is a fast one. In certain conditions the underlying cause of change in pH may have been treated, but if renal compensation has occurred, the end product of such compensation (for example, bicarbonate) will remain for several days after treatment (Tables 1 and 2).

TABLE 1. Examples of respiratory and metabolic acid-base disturbances

Acid-base disturbances	Causes	pH	Pa_{CO_2}	HCO_3^-	Mechanisms*
Acute respiratory acidosis	Alveolar hypoventilation	Decrease	Increase	Normal range	Increase in CO_2, thus H_2CO_3 and H^+; decrease in pH; no time for renal compensation
Chronic respiratory acidosis	Chronic alveolar hypoventilation	Normal range	Increase	Increase	Renal response to increase in CO_2: excrete more H^+; Results in reabsorption of $NaHCO_3$ to restore pH; increased HCO_3^-
Acute respiratory alkalosis	Alveolar hyperventilation	Increase	Decrease	Normal range	CO_2 "blown off," leaving less end products and excess of base; increased pH
Chronic respiratory alkalosis	Chronic alveolar hyperventilation	Normal range	Decrease	Decrease	Renal response to decreased CO_2: excrete more HCO_3^-, retain chloride to restore pH; hence less CO_2 and less HCO_3^-
Metabolic acidosis	Accumulation of (1) lactic acid in circulatory failure, (2) keto-acid in diabetes, or (3) inorganic acids in renal disease	Decrease	Decrease	Decrease	Addition of large amounts of fixed acids to blood results in loss of base (HCO_3^-) and decreased pH; immediate respiratory response results in decreased CO_2
Metabolic alkalosis	K^+ depletion, vomiting, diarrhea, $NaHCO_3$ excess or chloride depletion	Increase	Normal range or increase	Increase	Loss of acid or retention of base results in elevated pH and HCO_3^-; minimal respiratory response results in normal or elevated CO_2

*See text for explanations.

Respiratory and metabolic acid-base disturbances

An important fact to learn is that lung and renal function serve to maintain the proper pH by keeping the balance between CO_2 and HCO_3^-. Whatever acid or alkali is added to this system, the lungs and kidneys will continue to work to restore pH to normal. This is why compensated acid-base states occur. Acidosis or alkalosis may be respiratory or metabolic or mixtures of both. In Tables 1 and 2 some of these states are presented.

Normal values of pH and blood gases. A must in understanding blood gases and pH is to know the normal values. With electrode systems as they are today, there is no need for greater deviations than those presented here:

		Plasma		
pH	Pa_{CO_2}	HCO_3^- mEq/liter	Pa_{O_2}	O_2 Sat (S_{O_2})
7.38 to 7.42	38 to 42 mm Hg	23 to 25 mEq	95 to 100 mm Hg	97%

Another important factor to remember is that if pH is normal when arterial P_{CO_2} and/or bicarbonate is altered, *compensation* must have occurred or the acid-base abnormality is being treated.

TABLE 2. Possible causes of acid-base disturbances

Respiratory acidosis	Respiratory alkalosis

Primary factor: hypoventilation
  Pulmonary disease
  Drugs
  Obesity
  Mechanical asphyxia
  Sleep
	Primary factor: hyperventilation
	  Overventilation on a ventilator
	  Response to acidosis
	  Bacteremia
	  Thyrotoxicosis
	  Fever
	  Hepatic failure
	  Response to hypoxia
	  Hysteria

Metabolic acidosis	**Metabolic alkalosis**

Primary factor: addition of large amounts
  of fixed acids to body fluids
  Lactic acidosis (circulatory failure)
  Ketoacidosis (diabetes, starvation)
  Phosphates and sulfates (renal disease)
  Acid ingestion (salicylates)
  Secondary to respiratory alkalosis
  Adrenal insufficiency
	Primary factor: retention of base or
	  removal of acid from body fluids
	  Excessive gastric drainage
	  Vomiting
	  K^+ depletion (diuretic therapy)
	  Burns
	  Excessive $NaHCO_3$ administration

Respiratory acidosis. Alveolar hypoventilation *always* results in respiratory acidosis. This may be acute, chronic, or combined with metabolic processes. Patients with acute respiratory acidosis have an elevated arterial P_{CO_2} that causes an increase in H^+ and thus a decrease in pH. When the condition is acute, the kidneys will not have had time to compensate; therefore the bicarbonate level will be within normal range. The values for *acute respiratory acidosis* may be as follows:

pH 7.20 Pa_{CO_2} 60.0 mm Hg HCO_3^- 23.0 mEq/liter

The treatment for CO_2 retention is to remove it with adequate ventilation. It will not go away unless it is "blown off." If this condition goes untreated or becomes *chronic,* the values may be as follows:

pH 7.40 Pa_{CO_2} 60.0 mm Hg HCO_3^- 37.0 mEq/liter

The normal pH in this case shows that compensatory mechanisms have been at work to restore an equilibrium. The *retention* or *excretion* of HCO_3^- by the kidneys is dependent on PCO_2, and renal compensation in respiratory acidosis results from the reabsorption of HCO_3^- and the reduction of sodium excretion. This produces more $NaHCO_3$ for buffering. Additional free H^+ are excreted in the urine with chloride as HCl and ammonium chloride (NH_4Cl) so that electrical neutrality is maintained.

When renal compensation is complete,* the pH is normal because no free H^+ are present and conservation of HCO_3^- by the kidneys results in an elevated level of plasma bicarbonate. The preceding are typical acid-base values for patients with chronic obstructive airways disease who are "chronic" CO_2 retainers.

Acidosis may be primarily respiratory or be caused by a combination of respiratory and metabolic abnormalities. Alveolar hypoventilation always occurs, and there may be the addition of fixed acids; for example, there are ketones in diabetic acidosis and lactate in circulatory failure. Typical values for respiratory acidosis plus metabolic acidosis would be:

pH 7.20 Pa_{CO_2} 50.0 mm Hg HCO_3^- 19.0 mEq/liter

The pH is lower than normal, CO_2 is elevated, and HCO_3^- is slightly less than normal. Fixed acids cannot be blown off directly; they must be buffered. Bicarbonate plays an important role in this process and becomes depleted gradually without restoring pH.

This combined acid-base state is common in cardiac failure where metabolic acidosis and alveolar hypoventilation occur simultaneously.

Mixed acid-base states are not always easy to interpret. In the previous examples the HCO_3^- values were based on *actual* HCO_3^-, which is the bicarbonate concentration in plasma of an anaerobically drawn arterial blood sample. It is known from this how much bicarbonate is present in blood but not how much is present as a metabolic component or respiratory component.

Standard bicarbonate values in milliequivalents per liter tell us what the bicarbonate level would be if the blood were equilibrated at a normal PCO_2 (40 mm Hg).

---

*Rarely is renal compensation complete enough to restore pH to absolute normal, but it will restore pH to well within normal range.

From this the respiratory and metabolic component of acid-base status may be ascertained. Nomograms designed for this purpose are available.

Respiratory acidosis may also be accompanied by *metabolic alkalosis* caused by chloride deficiency or potassium deficiency. Electrical neutrality in red cells and plasma is not maintained because potassium is depleted and the kidneys are unable to excrete HCO_3^-. The HCO_3^- is added in excess because of the increased levels of CO_2. Typical values for respiratory acidosis plus metabolic alkalosis are:

$$\text{pH } 7.45 \quad Pa_{CO_2} \text{ 50.0 mm Hg} \quad HCO_3^- \text{ 35.0 mEq/liter}$$

pH in this case may be elevated or normal; Pa_{CO_2} is elevated because of hypoventilation; HCO_3^- is elevated excessively because of renal retention.

Respiratory alkalosis. Alveolar hyperventilation causes the reverse situation in which excess CO_2 is blown off, leaving less CO_2 available. Therefore less H^+ and HCO_3^- will be produced, the pH will be increased, and the Pa_{CO_2} value will be lowered. In *acute hyperventilation* the values may be:

$$\text{pH } 7.50 \quad Pa_{CO_2} \text{ 30.0 mm Hg} \quad HCO_3^- \text{ 24.0 mEq/liter}$$

Causes of respiratory alkalosis are neural response to hypoxia or acidosis by stimulation of respiratory centers, fever, hysteria, and overventilation by mechanical ventilators.

If respiratory alkalosis continues and becomes *chronic*, the kidneys excrete more bicarbonate and compensate by retaining chloride to restore both electrical neutrality and pH. Therefore, pH may be normal but with lower values for both Pco_2 and HCO_3^-:

$$\text{pH } 7.40 \quad Pa_{CO_2} \text{ 30.0 mm Hg} \quad HCO_3^- \text{ 18.0 mEq/liter}$$

Metabolic acidosis. Metabolic acidosis is caused by the accumulation of one or more of the "fixed" acids rather than carbonic acid. Clinically, the most common metabolic acidotic states are lactic acidosis from circulatory failure, ketoacidosis from diabetes, and inorganic acid accumulation of phosphates and sulfates in renal disease.

The normal distribution of anions and cations is thrown into imbalance as large amounts of a strong acid are added to plasma, with a massive increase in H^+. These acids are not blown off directly and therefore must be buffered.

Simple, acute metabolic acidosis with a normal Pco_2 rarely occurs. Usually respiratory compensation occurs at once, resulting in a decrease in Pco_2. Thus all the parameters of acid-base are *initially decreased:*

$$\text{pH } 7.20 \quad Pa_{CO_2} \text{ 30.0 mm Hg} \quad HCO_3^- \text{ 12.0 mEq/liter}$$

As body stores of HCO_3^- are reduced, pH-sensitive chemoreceptors in the neural pathway are stimulated and the response is hyperventilation.

A classic picture of metabolic acidosis is the panting, frightened patient who has a history of diabetes. When blood gases are analyzed, the following results may be seen:

$$\text{pH } 7.10 \quad Pa_{CO_2} \text{ 15.0 mm Hg} \quad HCO_3^- \text{ 5.0 mEq/liter}$$

Bicarbonate is used in increasing amounts in an attempt to restore pH, and as CO_2 is blown off, fewer end products ($H^+ + HCO_3^-$) are available from metabolism.

Neutralization of the acid present is the treatment for metabolic acidosis and restoration of anion-cation balance. (Metabolic acidosis and its treatment are discussed throughout the text with the disease states causing the condition. Special consideration is given to lactic acidosis in Chapter 9.)

Metabolic alkalosis. Metabolic alkalosis may be caused by depletion of potassium ions (K^+). This can occur from prolonged diuretic therapy, gastrointestinal disorders, or excessive gastric drainage. As H^+ and Cl^- decrease from loss of HCl, sodium becomes available to combine with bicarbonate, which increases levels of $NaHCO_3$. Excessive administration of $NaHCO_3$ has the same end result. Cellular K^+ depletion always leads to metabolic alkalosis with decreased levels of chloride. Alkalosis has a tendency to reduce respiratory drive, and thus carbon dioxide levels may be normal or elevated, whereas pH is elevated and HCO_3^- levels are above normal:

$$\text{pH } 7.50 \quad \text{Pa}_{CO_2} \text{ 45.0 mm Hg} \quad HCO_3^- \text{ 35.0 mEq/liter}$$

The interactions between electrolyte balance and carbon dioxide transport are far from simple in many disease states, and they are often further complicated by medical intervention. The examples presented illustrate the importance of carefully examining blood gas results along with other laboratory data. Blood gas values and pH are an integral part of patient management.

GUIDELINES IN SETTING POLICY FOR SAMPLING ARTERIAL BLOOD

Each hospital laboratory has its own set of guidelines to be used when arterial blood samples are to be obtained. A foundation for such guidelines is usually based on patient comfort during arterial puncture and on the quality of the sample obtained. The nurse may perform the arterial puncture or may be asked to assist. The ten guidelines that follow outline the principles involved when obtaining arterial blood samples.

1. Patient. As in any procedure the patient should be informed of what is going to happen to him. Special emphasis should be on normal quiet breathing whenever possible.

2. Equipment. When an arterial puncture is to be performed, the following equipment should be at hand: skin cleansing agents, sterile 5 to 10 ml glass syringes, heparin, a selection of needles, sterile gauze swabs, elastic strapping, labels, caps to seal the syringe, and a container of ice.

3. Skin preparation. Skin at the site of puncture should be thoroughly cleansed prior to arterial puncture. In some facilities aseptic technique is used (full skin preparation with a solution such as betadine, then sterile gloves worn by the person performing the puncture). Some physicians prefer the thorough use of two or three alcohol wipes to cleanse the skin.

Whatever method is used, fingers palpating an artery should also be clean. All too often medical staff don sterile gloves and then take a ballpoint pen to mark the position of the artery.

4. Site of puncture. Selection of the correct site for arterial puncture is a subject constantly debated by physicians. The final choice should, of course, be left to the patient's physician. Samples may be obtained from the radial, brachial, or femoral artery.

Hemostasis is easier in the smaller radial or brachial arteries than in the large femoral artery, and there are fewer anatomic structures to obscure the vessel. Pressure in the femoral vein is high, and a venous sample is often obtained by mistake when the femoral site is used.

5. Local anesthetic. Another subject of debate is the use of local anesthetic prior to arterial puncture. Some physicians can perform an arterial puncture without the use of local anesthetic, with no discomfort to the patient. Patient comfort and the quality of a blood sample often go hand in hand. If a patient is subjected to pain during an arterial puncture, the blood gas results will reflect this in the form of acute hyperventilation. A local anesthetic at the site of arterial puncture serves three purposes. First, it reduces pain and prevents unnecessary hyperventilation. Second, the bolus of local anesthetic on both sides of a vessel will prevent the vessel from rolling during puncture. Third, infiltration around the artery will reduce arterial spasm.

The argument against the use of local anesthetic is usually that a patient has to have two "sticks" instead of one when anesthetic is used. This would be a valid argument if a sample were always obtained during the first attempt. A local anesthetic, when given in sufficient quantity and allowed time to work, will eliminate discomfort should second or third attempts be made to obtain arterial blood.

6. Technique. Once the artery has been selected, careful palpation to ascertain position of the vessel should be carried out before puncture is attempted. Correct positioning of the arm will facilitate this. For puncture of the brachial artery, the arm should be fully extended and supported at the elbow with a firm towel roll or small sponge pillow. A rolled towel is placed under the wrist when the radial artery is used, and the hand is pushed down and back to obtain wrist extension (Fig. 5-4). An area of skin around the vessel is cleaned, position of the artery is checked, and local anesthetic is injected intradermally to numb the patient's skin before full infiltration.

A sterile 5 ml *heparinized* glass syringe fitted with a needle of wide bore (19 to 20 gauge), which will allow the free flow of blood into the syringe, should be used. Heparinization is achieved by drawing 0.5 ml of heparin (1:1,000) into the syringe and wetting the entire barrel by moving the plunger up and down the barrel. Excess heparin is carefully ejected, leaving the syringe free of *any* air bubbles and the needle filled with heparin. This prevents clotting of the sample.

With the syringe held at its base in one hand and the artery between the first and second fingers of the free hand (Fig. 5-5), the skin is entered with a firm, definite single puncture. The needle is advanced and then pulled back steadily. Once the artery is punctured, blood enters the syringe by fairly rapid pulsatile flow. When 3 to 5 ml of blood have been obtained, pressure should be applied above the artery with a folded piece of sterile gauze and the needle removed. The sample should be handed to a second person. Pressure must be applied for a full 5 minutes (longer if the patient

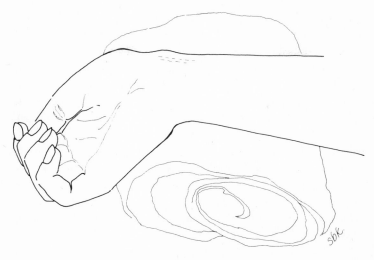

FIG. 5-4. Correct position to obtain wrist extension for puncture of the radial artery. Broken line approximates location of radial artery.

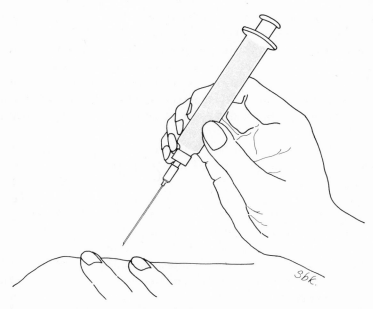

FIG. 5-5. Technique for puncture of the radial artery. Note the syringe is held at its base and the fingers of the free hand stabilize the artery.

is receiving anticoagulants) followed by application of a nonobstructing elastic pressure bandage.

7. Handling the sample. When the sample is obtained in the preceding manner, *aspiration is not necessary*, and no air bubbles should be present. Should air be introduced accidentally into a sample, it should be eliminated at once. With the sample held horizontally the needle is removed, and a cap is placed on the metal tip of the syringe to seal it. Then, by rotating the syringe, blood and heparin are mixed together to prevent clotting.

The sample should be placed in ice as soon as possible after collection (to slow down oxygen metabolism). The sample, correctly labeled with the patient's name, time of collection, patient's temperature, and PI_{O_2}, is then delivered to the blood gas laboratory.

8. Why is arterial blood used? Arterial blood is preferred (and many physicians believe it is essential) when measuring blood gases because it demonstrates what is going on in the lungs. Levels of oxygen in venous blood vary from organ to organ and limb to limb and do not provide information on the adequacy of ventilation, the degree of hypoxia, or the effectiveness of oxygen therapy.

The acid-base components are more accurate in arterial blood, and since arterial blood is essential for measuring oxygen, the other measurements can be made at the same time.

Micro blood-gas analyzers facilitate the use of arterialized capillary samples from small infants (such as premature infants) for measurement of pH and P_{CO_2}, but accuracy of oxygen measurements by this method is questionable.

9. Why is the patient's temperature important? Instruments used for analysis of blood gases are usually immersed in a thermostatically controlled water bath at 37° or 38° C. Since it would be impractical to change the water bath temperature to that of the patient each time a sample is analyzed, measurements are generally done under the preceding conditions and the results corrected to the patient's temperature. Arterial P_{O_2} and CO_2 increase with an increase in temperature and decrease with a decrease in temperature. The change in arterial P_{O_2} is about *6% for each centigrade degree change*.

Patients who are febrile or who are being nursed under hypothermic conditions often have marked deviations from normal body temperature, which will greatly affect final blood gas results. The following is an example of the importance of temperature.

Blood gas analysis is order for a patient at 11 AM, and the Pa_{O_2} is found to be 60 mm Hg. The 6 AM temperature of the patient (36° C) is given to the laboratory personnel, and this lowers the Pa_{O_2} to 54 mm Hg. However, the patient's actual temperature at 11 AM was 38° C, which would make the correct value 68 mm Hg.

Small differences such as these may appear insignificant, but if the values are borderline, the patient may be given oxygen unnecessarily, thus causing added cost and worry to the patient.

Patients nursed under conditions of hypothermia, where body temperature is considerably lower than normal, show differences from 50 to 100 mm Hg between the measured Pa_{O_2} and the actual Pa_{O_2} corrected for temperature. This becomes a critical factor when physiologic shunts are to be calculated (Chapter 11).

10. Why is PI_{O_2} important? When patients are receiving oxygen, it is important to know what the partial pressure of inspired oxygen is so that the effectiveness of O_2 therapy can be ascertained. Samples of inspired oxygen from the various types of equipment used for O_2 administration may be obtained and analyzed so that the exact O_2 delivery to patients is known and the accuracy of each delivery system is checked.

The normal concentration of oxygen in inspired air is 20.94%, which exerts a partial pressure of 149.3 mm Hg. This is calculated using the following method:

$$P = \frac{\text{gas concentration}}{100} \times P_B$$

This takes into account the water vapor pressure exerted at body temperature, 37° C. The equation reads as follows:

$$PI_{O_2} = \frac{20.94 \times (760 - 47)}{100} = 149.3 \text{ mm Hg}$$

This simple equation can be used to calculate any percentage of inspired oxygen, or fractional concentration (FI_{O_2}), and bring it to millimeters of mercury, in which the arterial Po_2 is reported.

The following examples illustrate what the PI_{O_2} would be with a patient receiving 100% O_2 and 50% O_2:

$$PI_{O_2} = \frac{100 \times (760 - 47)}{100} = 713 \text{ mm Hg}$$

and

$$PI_{O_2} = \frac{50 \times (760 - 47)}{100} = 356 \text{ mm Hg}$$

When patients are given 100% oxygen, one would expect the alveolar oxygen level to be the same as that inspired, 713 mm Hg. Carbon dioxide, however, exerts a partial pressure of 40 mm Hg, and oxygen consumption is a continuous process; hence, the normal values for arterial Po_2 in a patient receiving 100% O_2 are 580 to 620 mm Hg. This rise in Pa_{O_2} is normally possible because all the nitrogen in the lungs is washed out when 100% O_2 is delivered to patients with normal lungs.

PI_{O_2} can also be important in cases in which a set of blood gas results are in question. For example, a patient who is receiving 40% O_2 has stable vital signs and shows no obvious signs of deterioration; yet the arterial Po_2 is found to be 100 mm Hg when earlier in the day it was 180 mm Hg. Before any steps are taken to change settings on equipment in this situation, nurses should ask themselves four questions:

1. Is the patient really receiving 40% O_2; if so, was he receiving it when the blood sample was obtained?
2. How long had the patient been on 40% O_2 *before* blood gas analysis?
3. Has there been a laboratory error?
4. Has the condition of the patient changed?

Question 1 could have been eliminated had PI_{O_2} been measured at the time of blood gas analysis. In answer to question 2, patients should receive oxygen *continuously* for 20 to 30 minutes before arterial PO_2 measurements are taken for results to be accurate.

Should a physician want to know how high a patient can raise his arterial PO_2 when receiving 40% or 60% O_2, for example, it is of no value to deliver oxygen for 5 minutes to a patient and then obtain a sample. It takes time for oxygen levels to rise in blood because all areas of the lung are not ventilated and perfused evenly during normal quiet breathing.

When questions 1 and 2 are eliminated as reasons for an unusual change in arterial PO_2, question 3 may be asked because there is, of course, the possibility of laboratory error, which may account for the difference. Should this not be the case, the patient's condition should be reevaluated.

This simple process of elimination, particularly in questions 1 and 2, may save a patient the expense of having another arterial puncture. It is up to the nursing staff to make sure that patients receive the amount of oxygen ordered, for the correct amount of time before blood gas analysis, and to see that the *true* inspired oxygen concentration is known.

REFERENCES

Adams, A. P., Morgan-Hughes, J. O., and Sykes, M. K.: pH and blood-gas analysis: methods of measurement and sources of error using electrode systems, Anaesthesia **22:**575-597, 1967; **23:**47-64, 1968.

Bedford, R. F., and Wollman, H.: Complications of percutaneous radial artery cannulation; an objective prospective in man, Anesthesiology **38:**228-236, 1973.

Davenport, H. W.: The ABC of acid-base chemistry, ed. 5, Chicago, 1971, The University of Chicago Press.

Guyton, A. C.: Textbook of medical physiology, ed. 5, Philadelphia, 1976, W. B. Saunders Co.

Keyes, J. L.: Blood-gas analysis and the assessment of acid-base status, Heart Lung **5:**247-255, 1976.

Lambertsen, C. J.: Transport of oxygen and carbon dioxide by the blood. In Mountcastle, V. B., editor: Medical physiology, part V, vol. I, ed. 13, St. Louis, 1974, The C. V. Mosby Co.

Nunn, J. F.: Applied respiratory physiology, New York, 1969, Appleton-Century-Crofts.

Robertson, K. J., and Guzzetta, C. E.: Arterial blood-gas interpretations in the respiratory intensive care unit, Heart Lung **5:**256-260, 1976.

Shapiro, B. A.: Clinical application of blood gases, Chicago, 1973, Year Book Medical Publishers, Inc.

Snider, G. L.: Clinical interpretations of blood gases, Audiographic Series, Chicago, 1973, American College of Chest Physicians.

Wade, J. F.: Clinical correction of blood gas abnormalities (tape cassette), Anaheim, 1976, National Critical Care Institute of Education.

6 / CLASSIFICATION AND EVALUATION OF RESPIRATORY DISEASES

It is far beyond the scope of this text to present a detailed account of every disease entity associated with the respiratory system. I have selected those disorders most commonly encountered in hospital practice and hope that the reader will be stimulated to read the many fine works available on this subject (see chapter references).

Respiratory diseases are classified physiologically into two main groups—obstructive diseases and restrictive diseases (Table 3). *Obstructive* diseases are those respiratory diseases that obstruct the pathway of normal alveolar ventilation, either by spasm of the airways, mucus secretions, or morphopathologic changes of airways and/or alveoli. *Restrictive* diseases are those respiratory diseases that restrict movement of the thorax and/or lungs and may be associated with pathologic or neurologic factors.

OBSTRUCTIVE DISEASES

Three of the most common and serious obstructive diseases encountered in clinical medicine today are (1) chronic bronchitis, (2) pulmonary emphysema, and (3) bronchial asthma.

Chronic obstructive pulmonary disease (COPD) is a term often applied to those physiologic disorders associated with any or all of the preceding conditions. For example, a patient with chronic bronchitis may also have pulmonary emphysema and a bronchial asthmatic component to his disease, further complicated by cor pulmonale.

Although separate and distinct diseases, chronic bronchitis and pulmonary emphysema are found so frequently in the same patient that the term *bronchitis-emphysema syndrome* has developed. There are patients who have pure emphysema or pure chronic bronchitis, but many patients have the combined disorder.

Epidemiology. In industrial areas in the United Kingdom chronic respiratory disease (particularly bronchitis) has long been a condition that has hospitalized wage-earning males from 1 to 4 months during each winter, year after year. This is so much the rule rather than the exception that "winter bronchitis" is (sadly) an everyday phrase. My own experience in nursing patients with this disease in England taught me much of the physical, mental, and financial distresses wrought by it.

The increase in chronic bronchitis and emphysema in the United States has been rapid, and the National Center for Health Statistics reveals a continuing upward

TABLE 3. Obstructive and restrictive pulmonary diseases

Obstructive pulmonary diseases	Prime physiologic mechanisms
Chronic bronchitis	Expiratory airflow obstructed by excessive bronchial mucus secretion and pathologic changes in the airways
Pulmonary emphysema	Air "trapped" in overdistended alveoli; collapse of respiratory bronchioles on expiration causing prolongation of expiratory airflow
Bronchial asthma	Obstruction of expiratory airflow due to pathologic changes in airways, mucus plugs and spasms of smooth muscle.
Mucoviscidosis (cystic fibrosis)	Airways obstruction on expiration due to secretions and exudate
Coal miners' pneumoconiosis	Excessive bronchial secretion resulting in obstructed expiratory airflow

Restrictive pulmonary diseases	
Group classifications	Examples of disease entities
Neuromuscular disorders	Myasthenia gravis Poliomyelitis Guillain-Barré syndrome
Thoracic deformity	Kyphoscoliosis Pectus excavatum
Restriction to lung and/or alveolar expansion	Pneumothorax Pleural effusion Pulmonary fibrosis Pulmonary edema Atelectasis
Infiltrative diseases	Tuberculosis Carcinoma
Obesity	Pickwickian syndrome Abdominal ascites

trend in mortality from COPD, particularly emphysema. The latest available data show an increase of 12% in the number of deaths attributed to emphysema from 1964 to 1974. At this rate many of the hospital beds are going to be occupied in the years to come by patients with chronic respiratory disorders.

Chronic bronchitis and emphysema are often totally disabling. Respiratory cripples in the United States during 1973 were paid $400 million in Social Security payments. This amounted to 7.2% of all disability payments and is second only to those for heart disease.

The alarming increase in chronic bronchitis and emphysema not only in the United States but also in Japan, France, and many other countries has promoted an all-out effort at national and international levels for research into and control of these diseases.

Predisposing factors to chronic bronchitis and emphysema. The reader should keep in mind that two separate disease entities are being discussed here and that the pathology of each is different. Certain predisposing factors, however, appear to be common to both chronic bronchitis and emphysema:

1. Smoking
2. Atmospheric pollution
3. Climate
4. Occupation
5. Aging

Smoking. It is now well established by numerous studies and surveys that cigarette smoking is a most dangerous form of personal pollution. Despite the ban on cigarette advertising on television and radio and warnings by the National Heart Association, the U.S. Department of Health, Education and Welfare, the American Cancer Society, and the American Lung Association, the incidence of cigarette smoking is on the increase. It appears, too, that nonsmokers in the same room as smokers suffer some effects of cigarette pollutants.

Cigarette smoke is a complex chemical substance containing many carcinogenic substances. It is a constant irritant to the linings of the upper and lower respiratory tract and has a marked effect on the cardiovascular system.

The Surgeon General's Advisory Committee on Smoking and Health in 1964 determined that cough, sputum production, and reduction in ventilatory function occur more frequently in cigarette smokers. At that time it was stated that cigarette smoking is the single most important cause of chronic bronchitis and that it increases the risk of dying from the disease. In 1967, with the accumulation of more data, the conclusions of the report were strengthened and it was determined that cigarette smoking is the most important cause of chronic non-neoplastic bronchopulmonary disease in the United States and that it greatly increases the risk of dying from either chronic bronchitis or pulmonary emphysema.

Carbon monoxide is inhaled from cigarette smoke, and between 3% and 12% of available hemoglobin is chemically bound to it as carboxyhemoglobin. This reduces the amount of hemoglobin available to combine with and carry oxygen.

Cigarette smoke contains many carcinogenic agents and is a known contributory factor to malignant tumors of the larynx and thoracic cavity. Carcinogenic substances in cigarette smoke have a way of migrating from the respiratory tract into the stomach and bladder, which increases the incidence of malignancy in these organs in smokers.

Tobacco smoke insults the cardiovascular system by increasing the heart rate and producing vasoconstriction. The result is increased cardiac work to overcome the increased intravascular resistance (Chapter 4).

One of the serious effects of continuous tobacco inhalation is interference with the normal protective mechanisms of the lungs; these include mucus production, ciliary activity, and phagocytic activity.

Because of the constant irritation to the epithelium lining the airways, cigarette smoke increases activity of the mucus-secreting goblet cells and the mucus glands of the membrane propria. The excess mucus produced must be removed, which puts a burden on ciliary activity. A vicious cycle is then set up because cigarette smoke also inhibits ciliary activity; thus movement of the mucociliary blanket is slowed or stopped. Particulate matter and bacteria are not readily removed, and the result is inflammation and infection. Long-term effects are the pathologic changes seen in the airways and alveoli in chronic bronchitis and emphysema.

Many of the respiratory changes brought about by the inhalation of cigarette smoke are reversible over a period of time after discontinuation of cigarette smoking. Studies of pulmonary function on ex-smokers show improvement in ventilatory function 5 years after tobacco smoke inhalation ceases. This is not the case, however, if destructive emphysematous changes have occurred.

Nurses can do much to educate the public in the dangers of tobacco inhalation by keeping up on current health statistics associated with the subject and relaying this information to friends and relatives.

Atmospheric pollution. The subject of atmospheric pollution is one that has provided much dinner conversation for many Americans. It has also become, in its relationship to disease, a main topic at conferences in major industrial cities throughout the world. The United Nations, at its first conference on human environment, proposed setting up a worldwide network of a hundred stations to monitor air pollution.

There now appears to be little doubt concerning the effects of atmospheric pollutants on persons with or without respiratory disease. In London during December, 1952, a severe episode of air pollution resulted in a massive increase in mortality in patients with chronic respiratory disease. Some 4,000 deaths occurred within a few days. In New York in 1966 a similar increase in atmospheric pollution also brought about a rise in the mortality of such patients.

A large percentage of atmospheric pollutants result from the exhaust emissions of automobiles and from industry. The composition and concentration of atmospheric pollutants vary from area to area depending on the types of industry in those areas and the number of automotive vehicles.

The main components of atmospheric pollutants are sulfur dioxide (SO_2), nitrogen dioxide (NO_2), ozone (O_3), carbon monoxide (CO), and many hydrocarbons.

Climate. A combination of cold and dampness appears to contribute to recurrence of chronic bronchitis. The cold, damp winters in the British Isles result in a marked increase in upper and lower respiratory tract infections.

Occupation. Occupations that expose persons to dust particles (for example, in mining and carpentry) are thought to increase the incidence of bronchitis-emphysema syndrome. Exposure to high concentrations of nitrous dioxide and sulfur dioxide gases is also thought to be a cause.

Many other respiratory diseases are closely correlated with occupation and exposure to chemicals. Some of these diseases include silicosis, asbestosis, and pneumoconiosis. Past and present occupations of the patient may provide a clue to his disease entity.

Aging. The aging process reduces the normal elastic qualities of lung tissue and the thoracic cage. Changes in the shape of the spine increase the anteroposterior diameter of the chest and give the thorax a kyphotic appearance. Because of loss of alveolar elasticity, there is some hyperinflation of alveoli in the aging lung. These factors were thought to contribute to the changes seen in pulmonary emphysema, and many studies have been conducted to prove this. However, the important difference between the aging process and pulmonary emphysema is that the aging process occurs in males and females and smokers and nonsmokers, whereas pulmonary emphysema is essentially a disease of older males with a history of cigarette smoking. The lungs' aging process does not normally restrict everyday activity, whereas pulmonary emphysema is a disabling disease. Pathologic changes in the lungs are more pronounced and destructive in pulmonary emphysema than in the aging lung.

Miscellaneous factors. Many other factors are thought to predispose a person to chronic bronchitis and pulmonary emphysema. Some are sex, genetics, race, allergy, and infection. The bronchitis-emphysema syndrome occurs much more frequently in males than females. Whites are thought to be much more susceptible than blacks, although some studies show that with a similar smoking history and environment the difference between the groups is not significant. A genetic deficiency in a serum protein known as alpha$_1$-antitrypsin is related to a type of familial emphysema that occurs mainly in women.

Pulmonary emphysema

The etiology of pulmonary emphysema is essentially unknown; however, the predisposing factors just described are known to be contributory. The etiology is vague because of the difficulty in producing the disease in laboratory animals. Pulmonary emphysema appears to be mainly a disease of the Caucasian urban male. The experimental difficulty is compounded because of the differences in lung architecture between animal species and humans. A similar disease occurs in horses, and emphysematous changes have been effected in tracheostomized dogs after continuous inhalation of cigarette smoke.

Pulmonary emphysema was first described by the French physician Laennec in 1820, but a clear and widely accepted definition of the disease was not formulated until 1960. It is now clear that pulmonary emphysema is a destructive disease involving the gas exchanging areas of the lungs and is best described by the pathologic changes that follow.

Pathology. The pathologic changes in pulmonary emphysema cause the two distinctive features of the disease: (1) The elastic tissue of alveolar walls and alveolar septa is destroyed and (2) there is loss of alveolar tone and hyperinflation of affected alveoli. This blowing out or overinflation of alveoli is usually accompanied by retention, or trapping, of alveolar air.

There are two types of pulmonary emphysema, which occur either together or separately. *Centrilobular* (centriacinar) emphysema, as the name implies, occurs anatomically in the central portion of the lobule close to respiratory bronchioles (Chapter 1). The disease is often seen in patients 40 to 50 years of age and is frequently associated with chronic bronchitis. As the disease progresses, destruction of the lobule occurs from the center outward until the whole lobule becomes a big air space, or *bulla. Panlobular* (panacinar) emphysema is more generalized and occurs in the acinar units with destruction of alveolar septa and walls. This type of emphysema is more common in older males (60 to 70 years of age). Chronic bronchitis is less frequent in panlobular emphysema. As the disease progresses, destruction of the pulmonary capillary bed accompanies alveolar destruction.

Clinical manifestations. Unfortunately, pulmonary emphysema is an insidious disease, and unless an individual is active there may be no symptoms until 20% to 30% of the lung tissue has been destroyed. Dyspnea on exertion is one of the first complaints that will bring an individual to seek medical help.

The patient with pulmonary emphysema is generally an older, emaciated male with much muscle wasting. A characteristic increase in the anteroposterior diameter of the chest is usually seen, which gives a "barrel" chest appearance. Curvature of the spine, such as is present in kyphosis, is often observed but may be due to aging.

On further examination many of the compensatory respiratory mechanisms that the patient has adopted over the years will be noted. One of these is the extremely prolonged *expiratory* phase of respiration through pursed lips. Because of loss of elastic qualities of lung tissue, the minute respiratory and terminal bronchioles tend to collapse when the patient exhales at normal speed. But by letting his air out slowly through pursed lips, the patient can reduce this collapsing mechanism and thus exhale more completely.

As the disease progresses, the patient with emphysema uses all his accessory muscles of respiration in order to breathe. The shoulder girdle is elevated and the thorax tends to move up and down rather than in and out.

The patient's history usually reveals that he has been a heavy cigarette smoker most of his life. Cough will generally be denied except for what the patient may term his "smoker's" cough. The patient with pulmonary emphysema has a chronic hacking cough, which is so much a part of his existence that to him it is unimportant. Sputum production in emphysema in its pure form is usually slight and mucoid in character. In the presence of bronchitis, copious amounts of thick mucopurulent sputum is expectorated.

Even in the presence of severe disease, the patient with pulmonary emphysema maintains normal gas exchange and often has an elevated hematocrit value. This gives the patient a "pink and puffy" appearance compared with the cyanotic appearance of the person with chronic bronchitis.

Changes in pulmonary function. The patient with pulmonary emphysema demonstrates many changes in his pulmonary function status. When a patient is asymptomatic, the early detection of disease changes is often possible through pulmonary function testing.

Lung volumes. Because the alveoli are hyperinflated, pulmonary emphysema is characterized by an increase in residual volume, which results in an increase in functional residual capacity and in total lung capacity (Chapter 3). As emphysema progresses, a reduction in vital capacity occurs because of the loss of lung parenchyma and musculoelastic properties, which prevents a maximal inspiration or expiration.

When vital capacity is reduced and residual volume increased, the result is still a normal total lung capacity even in the presence of severe disease.

Mechanics. Normally a person can force out all his air (FEV) in 3 seconds. But because of severe air trapping, increased airways resistance, and collapse of respiratory bronchioles during expiration, it may take the patient with emphysema up to 20 to 30 seconds. I find it rather sad that patients who keep forcing out air over several seconds believe that because they can keep going so long their lungs are really very healthy.

All rates of flow are reduced, as is maximal voluntary ventilation, in the patient with emphysema. Unless there is pronounced bronchospasm present at the time of testing, there is no significant improvement seen in lung volumes or mechanics after administration of bronchodilator therapy.

Arterial blood gases. When pulmonary emphysema is present *without* chronic bronchitis, arterial blood gases may show a slight reduction in arterial Po_2 or may be normal. This seeming contradiction exists because alveolar destruction is accompanied by pulmonary capillary destruction; therefore the ventilation–to–blood flow relationship is maintained near normal.

As the disease progresses, alveolar hypoventilation may occur because of loss of mechanical properties of the thorax and muscular fatigue. The changes in blood gases would then be increased arterial Pco_2 and a decreased Pa_{O_2}.

Complications. Loss of pulmonary vasculature results in an increase in pulmonary vascular resistance, causing pulmonary hypertension and cor pulmonale. These features of the disease may not manifest themselves until late in the destructive process (for example, not until 70% of the lung tissue and vasculature has been destroyed). Alveolar hypoventilation and the related hypercapnia and hypoxemia predispose the patient to sudden respiratory failure. The patient with emphysema can become totally disabled; he may become a respiratory cripple who sits, fights for each breath, and wastes away—a pathetic figure to himself and to his family.

Medical and nursing management. A main objective in managing the patient with emphysema is to provide enough rehabilitation to restore him to a level of activity that will enable him to be a more useful person. This requires team effort involving patient, family, medical, nursing, and paramedical cooperation. Pulmonary emphysema cannot be cured, but much can be done to alleviate some of the misery wrought by the disease.

The first part of an emphysema rehabilitation program involves mental rehabilitation. Cigarette smoking should be stopped, and in a hospital room in the presence of oxygen a no-smoking rule is easily enforced. This is not always the answer to a lifelong, deeply entrenched habit. The patient must want to stop smoking and must do so if any rehabilitation program is going to succeed. Psychiatric counseling may be necessary in order to help the patient with emphysema to overcome his desire to smoke and foster a desire to improve his health. A busy but nonexhausting rehabilitation day-care plan is of great value in keeping patients away from their cigarette crutch. This should include nutrition, physical therapy, and occupational therapy.

Anorexia and weight loss are major problems that can be corrected by feeding the patient several small nutritious meals throughout the day rather than giving him three large meals. It is up to the nursing staff to see that nourishment is taken by the patient and to schedule other daily activities around the mealtimes so that the patient is not rushed.

Dyspnea on exertion as a major symptom is often relieved by oxygen-assisted exercise programs. Muscle wasting and lack of muscle tone are treated with physical therapy, which is conducted more easily if the patient inhales 2 to 3 liters of oxygen per minute by way of nasal cannula during the exercise periods.

Chronic bronchitis

The most accepted definition of chronic bronchitis is based on clinical findings: cough, sputum production, and a time factor. The patient with chronic bronchitis generally has recurrent, excessive, bronchial mucus secretion, resulting in a productive cough. The cough is found to occur on most days for at least 3 months of the year during at least 2 consecutive years.

Etiology. It is now clearly demonstrated that chronic bronchitis is caused by cigarette smoking and that the incidence is higher in urban industrial areas. Climate, occupation, and economics are also contributory factors.

Pathology. Hypertrophy of bronchial mucosal glands occurs in chronic bronchitis, accompanied by chronic inflammatory cell infiltration and edema of bronchial mucosa. The chronic cough in presence of increased bronchial secretions appears to affect the minute bronchioles to the point of total destruction. Slowing or loss of ciliary and phagocytic activity due to smoking and increased mucus secretion leaves the patient as a perfect host for bacteria.

Clinical manifestations. The patient with chronic bronchitis will usually seek medical aid as a result of shortness of breath associated with wheeze. Not uncommonly the symptoms will coincide with a recent respiratory infection. He will have a productive cough and will state that he expectorates large amounts of sputum, most of which is eliminated in the early morning. An audible wheeze is generally found, which is often heard along with coarse rales and rhonchi throughout both lung fields. In later stages of the disease sacral and ankle edema may be present, and neck veins may be distended because of right ventricular failure from long-standing pulmonary hypertension. Presence of cyanosis is often detected by examination of the nail beds and mucus membranes.

The description "blue and bloated" is assigned to the classic appearance of the pure bronchitic patient because of the presence of hypoxemia resulting in cyanosis and the tendency to edema in these patients.

When a history is taken from the patient, it will be found that he is in early middle age or younger, has smoked heavily during his entire adult life, and has a long history of recurrent chest infections often related to winter weather.

Changes in pulmonary function. Survey studies of pulmonary function have provided valuable information in the early detection of changes in the mechanical properties of the lung associated with atmospheric pollution and smoking. This is an important factor in the early detection of chronic bronchitis. For example, groups of school children have been studied in large industrial cities in England and results compared with similar groups studied in rural areas. The children from the industrial group were found to have much more mucus secretion than those of the rural area, which resulted in a reduction in their forced expiratory volume at 1 and 3 seconds.

Lung volumes. Because of pathologic changes in the airways (thickening), the patient with chronic bronchitis often has a *reduced vital capacity*. When no emphysematous changes are present, the residual volume will be normal.

Mechanics. All measurements of rates of flow are reduced. These include FEF200-1200, FEF25-75%, FIVC, FEV_1, and FEV_3 (Chapter 4). This reduction is caused by bronchial secretions and pathologic changes in the airways. Because of the likely occurrence of bronchospasm with chronic bronchitis, there may be a marked improvement in pulmonary mechanics following bronchodilator therapy. Sometimes, however, it is difficult to attribute all such improvement entirely to bronchodilators because of the large amounts of secretions cleared during pulmonary function testing.

When breathing tests are performed by these patients, the effect is one of exercise for the lungs and opening of airways and alveoli that are not normally ventilated.

Arterial blood gases. In chronic bronchitis, signs of alveolar hypoventilation are reflected in the blood gases as hypoxemia and hypercapnia. The reasons for the hypoventilation are not entirely know, but it appears to be a type of compensatory mechanism for the chronic bronchitic patient. Further physiologic complications from the low arterial Po_2 and the respiratory acidosis are vasoconstrictive, resulting in increased vascular resistance. There is an increase in pulmonary artery pressure and an increase in right ventricular work. This is the origin of cor pulmonale so often found as a development in patients with chronic bronchitis.

Complications. Many patients with chronic bronchitis develop pulmonary emphysema, which is compounded by the further complication of cor pulmonale. Acute respiratory failure may occur with any recurrent infection that increases secretion and worsens hypoventilation; more carbon dioxide accumulates and respiratory failure follows.

In addition to the physical complications, there are financial and social complications. Many patients with chronic bronchitis have poor work records because of working days lost because of illness. Loss of work, when added to a poor economic situation, increases patient and family suffering. The whole picture is extremely depressing.

Medical and nursing management. Only a brief overview of medical and nursing management will be presented at this time. The subject is discussed in more detail in Chapter 10.

The patients with chronic bronchitis with or without emphysema present a medical and nursing challenge. Often such patients are irritable as a result of hypoxemia and hypercapnia. They become easily discouraged with the nursing staff and their medical care; they often appear agitated and hostile.

A main objective of medical and nursing management is to improve alveolar ventilation and relieve hypoxemia. To improve alveolar ventilation, bronchial secretions must first be removed by rigorous pulmonary toilet accomplished through postural drainage and physical therapy. Intermittent positive pressure breathing (IPPB) therapy is used to aerate the alveoli, remove carbon dioxide, and deliver bronchodilator therapy and mucolytic agents.

Controlled oxygen therapy will relieve the hypoxemia. Serial blood gas analysis and tests of pulmonary function are used to evaluate the effectiveness of management.

Asthma

There are few nurses who have not seen a child or adult fighting for every breath—for life itself—during a severe attack of asthma. Approximately 8 million people in the United States are afflicted with asthma, and this serious respiratory disease carries a high mortality rate with it. In many instances an asthmatic attack will be unresponsive to conventional therapy and constitutes a life-threatening situation, known as *status asthmaticus.* As many as 3% of patients admitted to the hospital in status asthmaticus die from it. Treatment of this medical emergency is discussed in Chapter 10.

Asthma, as defined by the American Thoracic Society, is "a disease characterized by an increased responsiveness of the airways to various stimuli manifested by widespread narrowing of the airways that changes in severity either spontaneously or as a result of therapy." Although asthma frequently occurs in individuals who have a family history of allergies (hay fever, urticaria, or other allergic conditions), it also occurs in persons who have no family or personal history of any allergic conditions.

Asthma generally occurs intermittently, which means that the patient may be symptom free from episodes of bronchospasm for months or years.

Etiology. Asthma is a hyperresponsiveness of the airways to certain "triggering" mechanisms (irritants or allergens), which predispose several physiologic and pharmacologic events. The etiology of asthma remains essentially unknown, although there are several hypotheses. Two major areas of etiologic investigation have been (1) the antigen-antibody theory and (2) the role of the autonomic nervous system in the regulation of bronchial smooth muscle activity. Let us now look at these in turn.

An *antibody* is a protein, and antibodies are formed in the human body by lymphatics in response to invasion by a foreign substance, an *antigen.* In the lung of the person with asthma the antigen-antibody reaction is thought to occur in tissue mast cells (lying just beneath the bronchial epithelium) and possibly in some circulating basophils.

A special group of immunoglobulins, known as IgE, attach themselves or become bound to the mast cells. In response to an invading antigen (allergen), these cells become active and undergo the process of degranulation. As this occurs, certain enzymatic and pharmacologic substances are released: histamine and slow-reacting substance of anaphylaxis (SRS-A). Other chemical mediators, such as bradykinin, acetylcholine, serotonin and certain prostaglandins, are also thought to be involved in the preceding reaction.

The effect from release of these chemical substances is bronchoconstriction. Histamine release, in particular, leads to severe bronchospasm, significant increase in the production of mucus, and the development of localized bronchial swelling and edema.

It is known that asthma attacks in patients frequently occur nonimmunologically. For example, a deep breath of fresh cold morning air causes the patient with a hyperactive airway to have severe bronchospasm. Emotional stress, exercise, and irritants may also trigger an asthma attack. Both the sympathetic and the parasympathetic nervous systems appear to play a role in asthma: the sympathetic nervous system because of *adrenergic* activity involving alpha and beta receptors, and the parasympathetic system because of *cholinergic* activity and the vagus nerve.

In 1948 Dr. R. P. Ahlquist proposed that there were two types of adrenergic receptors, alpha and beta. During the 1960s the beta receptors were divided into two subgroups, beta-1 and beta-2. Beta-2 receptors are thought to be present in the glands, smooth muscle, and mucosal vessels of the bronchial tree. Adrenergic stimulation of beta-2 receptors results in bronchodilatation. The importance of the beta-2 receptors has led to considerable pharmacologic research in selecting a drug with direct and specific beta-2 stimulation for the treatment of asthma.

A diminished responsiveness of the beta-2 receptors to stimulation was suggested by Dr. Szentivanyi in 1958 as the underlying mechanism in asthma. This is the foundation for the beta-adrenergic blockade theory. When beta-2 response is decreased, the bronchial tree is extremely irritable and open to cholinergic (bronchoconstrictive) stimulation.

Nervous system involvement in asthma is best thought of in terms of neuropharmacology because of the complex chemical and hormonal sequence of events that occurs when an asthma attack is triggered. This is supported by a further hypothesis, which is particularly important to the management of the asthmatic patient: that the beta-2 receptor is an enzyme adenyl cyclase, which after adrenergic stimulation catalyzes the conversion of adenosine triphosphate (ATP) to the substance cyclic 3′-5′-adenosine monophosphate (cyclic AMP). It is known that cyclic AMP produces bronchodilatation.

The major principle behind effective bronchodilator therapy is either to stimulate production of cyclic AMP or to decrease its breakdown. This will be discussed further with bronchodilator drugs, in Chapter 9.

Pathology. One of the major pathologic findings in asthma is the occlusion of bronchi and bronchioles with thick, tenacious mucus plugs, which on examination are found to contain portions of the lining epithelium. Such plugs are often expectorated by the patient during or following an attack of asthma, and may actually resemble a fine branch of the bronchial tree.

The lining epithelium of bronchi and bronchioles becomes detached in the patient with asthma. The basement membrane (Chapter 1) is then left exposed, which results in its becoming inflamed and thickened. Spasm of smooth muscle of the airways is also present, which causes them to constrict. The narrowed and clogged airways prevent the passage of air through them. Air in the alveoli distal to the occlusion cannot escape and therefore is eventually absorbed by the blood, resulting in atelectasis of the affected alveoli.

The pathology of asthma demonstrates Poiseuille's law (Chapter 2). The narrowing of the airways and the presence of turbulent airflow result in increased airway resistance; therefore an increase in the work of breathing is required to move a volume of air through the airways.

Clinical manifestations. Asthma occurs in patients of all ages. Usually the history reveals that the patient has had recurrent attacks of wheezing, which are predisposed by exposure to an allergic factor. Night coughing and sputum production (particularly after an attack) also occur.

During an acute asthmatic attack, the patient will appear distressed and will fight for air. Wheezing is often audible from across the room. On examination, wheezes and ronchi are heard throughout the entire lung fields, and the expiratory phase of respiration is performed with great difficulty. Inspiratory rib retractions are evident.

Changes in pulmonary function. Patients with bronchial asthma show varying degrees of change in pulmonary function status depending on whether their disease is adequately controlled, in a period of remission, or in the period of an attack.

Lung volumes. The vital capacity may be severely reduced because of smooth muscle spasm and collection of secretions. Residual volume may be increased because of hyperinflation of alveoli caused by loss of elastic recoil and airway blockage.

Mechanics. Because of spasm with increased airways resistance, all flow rates (FEF200-1200, FEF25-75%, FIVC, FEV_1 and FEV_3) are greatly reduced. There is nothing quite as dramatic as the response to bronchodilator therapy seen in some patients during pulmonary function testing. FEV_1 and FEV_3 are often doubled and tripled, returning this part of pulmonary function to normal. An increase in vital capacity usually accompanies these changes following bronchodilator therapy.

Arterial blood gases. A reflection of inadequate alveolar ventilation (because of airways obstruction and microatelectasis) with respect to blood flow is demonstrated by a reduction in arterial Po_2. As the disease progresses, certain acid-base irregularities evolve. A rise in arterial carbon dioxide levels in the asthmatic patient is indicative of severe bronchospasm with a marked increase in the amount of wasted ventilation.

Complications. The major complication of asthma is loss of control of the disease state, where episodic attacks become more frequent and therapy less effective. If this situation progresses, status asthmaticus and respiratory failure follow.

Medical and nursing management. The main objective in management of the patient with asthma is to prevent recurrence of the attacks or to reduce their frequency. (The former, of course, is highly desirable but not always possible.) Isolation of the offending allergens and the prevention of any psychological factor that may predispose an attack is of great value in therapy.

Outpatient control with maintenance doses of a bronchodilator agent such as Tedral or terbutaline (Chapter 9) is advisable. Pocket nebulizers containing a bronchodilator such as isoproterenol are useful in controlling mild symptoms of an attack.

The patient admitted with the *acute asthmatic attack* demands the most of the nurse's skills. Patient fear and apprehension must be alleviated and the family comforted. Children are often the victims and are extremely apprehensive not only about the lack of air but also the hospital surroundings (Chapter 10).

RESTRICTIVE DISEASES

Many disease entities contribute to pulmonary restriction (Table 3) but all, through varying mechanisms, result in a reduction in the vital capacity and alter ventilatory function. Because most of the restrictive conditions bring about an overall reduction in compliance of the thorax and/or lung tissue, the result is loss of chest expansion and therefore a reduction in the volume of air inspired and expired.

Neuromuscular disorders

Patients suffering from myasthenia gravis, Guillain-Barré syndrome, or bulbar poliomyelitis are subject to varying degrees of alveolar hypoventilation because interference in neural conduction causes respiratory muscle weakness.

Myasthenia gravis. Myasthenia gravis is characterized by the development of generalized muscular weakness causing difficulty in swallowing, which prevents patients from managing their normal oral secretions. There is often a reduction in vital capacity. As the disease progresses, the vital capacity continues to decrease to the point where tracheostomy and mechanical ventilatory support may become necessary. Daily monitoring of the vital capacity in patients with myasthenia gravis is necessary to establish the effectiveness of any treatment given and to enable the medical staff to prepare the patient psychologically if the condition becomes severe enough to warrant ventilatory support.

Myasthenia gravis is caused by reduction of acetylcholine at myoneural junctions, and the diagnosis is readily confirmed by the administration of an acetylcholinesterase inhibitor, such as *edrophonium chloride (Tensilon)*. When given in a 5 mg dose intravenously to an untreated myasthenic patient, it will result in complete *temporary* relief of all symptoms.

Treatment in the less severe cases of myasthenia gravis with anticholinesterase agents such as *pyridostigmine (Mestinon)* results in effective relief of symptoms. This is accomplished by the drug inhibiting the breakdown of acetylcholine by the enzyme cholinesterase. Side effects of such drugs may result in a "cholinergic crisis," which is evident by excessive salivation, nausea, abdominal cramps, and muscular weakness. These toxic effects should be watched for, particularly if the drug dosage must be increased to control symptoms.

Guillain-Barré syndrome. Guillain-Barré syndrome is acute infectious polyneuritis and is characterized by headache, aching limbs, general malaise, and slight fever; these symptoms may be mistaken for influenza. As the disease progresses, a sensation of numbness and tingling in the fingers and toes may be noticed by the patient and is accompanied by varying degrees of muscular weakness and paralysis. These symptoms progress to involve the respiratory muscles, which results in respiratory embarrassment and the necessity for tracheostomy and mechanical ventilation.

Lumbar puncture and examination of the cerebrospinal fluid will reveal an increase in the protein content with no increase in cell count. This finding in conjunction with the above symptoms will usually confirm the diagnosis. In adults the symptoms of the Guillain-Barré syndrome may be more easily recognized than in young children. Parents may associate the symptoms in children with some other childhood ailment. (I have cared for two such children, 5 and 8 years of age, for whom a prompt emergency room diagnosis and medical intervention were life saving.)

Bulbar poliomyelitis. Bulbar poliomyelitis is a virus infection involving the 9th to 12th cranial nerves. It affects the pharynx (hence swallowing) and results in paralysis of the laryngeal muscles. The patient may have voice changes and as the disease progresses, will aspirate secretions. A second type of poliomyelitis, the spinal type, affects the muscles of respiration causing weakness and eventually failure. Patients with bulbar poliomyelitis are often tracheostomized in order to manage their secretions; patients with spinal poliomyelitis are nursed in tank ventilators. Fortunately, poliomyelitis occurs much less frequently than formerly because of widespread immunization.

Thoracic deformity

Restriction to chest expansion caused by alteration in the structure and shape of the thorax may also affect expansion of the lungs within. This may be from kyphoscoliosis (an abnormal convex curvature of the spine) or pectus excavatum (funnel chest, a concave deformity caused by depression of the sternum). Both conditions cause a decrease in vital capacity. Patients with kyphoscoliosis may have severe limitation to ventilatory function, which leaves them host to respiratory complications following a chest infection, such as pneumonia, or after surgery. In clinical practice restriction to thoracic expansion may be induced by tight strapping, surgical incisions of the thorax, or pain.

Restriction to lung and/or alveolar expansion

Conditions that restrict the expansion of the lungs and/or alveoli reduce the vital capacity and the volume of air available for gas exchange. This may result from compression of the lung from within the thorax, by fluid, blood, pus or air, collections of fluid at the alveolar level, or collapsed alveoli.

Spontaneous pneumothorax. Introduction of air into the intrapleural space results in spontaneous pneumothorax (Chapter 1), which may be caused by trauma to the chest wall, rupture of alveoli as in emphysematous bullae, or infiltrative lesions of the lung. The result is partial or total collapse of the lung on the affected side, expansion of the thoracic cage on the affected side, and a shift in mediastinal contents toward the *unaffected* side. Patients with a pneumothorax will complain of dyspnea, an irritating cough, and chest pain. For reexpansion of the affected lung to take place, the negative intrapleural pressure should be reestablished. This is accomplished by sealing the air leak and by the application of suction using an underwater seal drainage system.

Pleural effusion. Pleural effusion is a collection of fluid (transudate or exudate) in the pleural cavity, which compresses lung tissue and thereby interferes with normal ventilaton. Pulmonary diseases such as tuberculosis, pneumonia, pleurisy, and carcinoma may be predisposing factors and the condition not infrequently recurs. The underlying cause of the condition must be treated. Fluid is removed from the pleural space by thoracentesis, which serves the dual purpose of relieving compression of the lung and providing a specimen of pleural fluid for laboratory examination.

Other conditions where changes in the pleural space may cause lung compression and/or interfere with respiratory function include hydrothorax, hemothorax, fibrothorax, and empyema.

Hydrothorax. Hydrothorax is an accumulation of serous fluid in the pleural space. It is caused by fluid being forced into the pleural cavity because of severe venous congestion in congestive heart failure, by blockage of a major lymphatic vessel, or by hepatic cirrhosis.

Hemothorax. Hemothorax, a pooling of free blood in the pleural space, is usually caused by trauma such as crush injuries to the chest.

Fibrothorax. Fibrothorax, where the visceral and parietal pleurae are adherent to each other, results in a thick, tight, nonexpansible skin around the affected lung. This causes loss of function and respiratory impairment. The development of fibrothorax usually follows insult to the pleurae by repeated tuberculous pleural effusions or by other conditions affecting the pleura. Decortication, or peeling, of the fibrotic layer off the lung is often effective in improving ventilatory function.

Pulmonary fibrosis. Pulmonary fibrosis is a diffuse interstitial disease of the lung, which results in a marked decrease in lung compliance and a diffusion defect. It may be predisposed by certain occupational diseases (silicosis, asbestosis) or collagen diseases or radiation therapy. In many instances the cause of the disease is unknown, and a group of such disorders is known as the Hamman-Rich syndrome.

Infiltrative diseases

Restriction to pulmonary ventilation occurs in infiltrative diseases because of damage to healthy lung tissue through invasion of the respiratory system by bacteria, irritants, or malignant cells. This can result in chronically inflamed lung tissue, producing scarring, loss of lung compliance, and impairment of respiratory function.

Pulmonary tuberculosis. Pulmonary tuberculosis results from invasion of the respiratory system by the tubercle bacillus, *Mycobacterium tuberculosis*. The tubercle bacilli are transmitted through the air and are usually inhaled. An inflammation is then set up, and the tubercular lesion in the lung may persist as granuloma, may progress through caseation to tissue necrosis, or may heal as a scar. In the early stages of pulmonary tuberculosis the patient is often asymptomatic; as the disease progresses, malaise, fatigue, weight loss, cough, and hemoptysis will bring the patient to seek medical aid. A treatment regimen includes bedrest with isolation precautions, mental relaxation, and drug therapy.

Principal drugs used in the treatment of pulmonary tuberculosis are isoniazid (INH), para-aminosalicylic acid (PAS), ethambutol (EMB), streptomycin, and rifampin. Ethambutol is frequently used in place of PAS in combination with INH and streptomycin. Rifampin, one of the newer antibiotics in the treatment of pulmonary tuberculosis, is being used in place of streptomycin in combination therapy.

Bronchogenic carcinoma. Bronchogenic carcinoma is so called because primary neoplastic lesions of the lung commonly arise in the mucous membranes of the bronchial tree. The lung is also the most common site for metastases from neoplasms located elsewhere in the body. The disease occurs predominately in men (5 to 1) and is closely related to the number of cigarettes smoked each day. The death rate from lung cancer is nine times as high for smokers as for nonsmokers, and for those who smoke two packs a day it is twenty times as high. The number of deaths from lung cancer in the United States is approaching 84,000 per year, compared with about 49,000 in 1968.

Respiratory impairment results from infiltration and destruction of lung tissue by malignant cells and invasion of the ribs and mediastinal structures. Bronchogenic carcinoma has an insidious onset, and symptoms such as cough and wheeze may go unnoticed or be attributed to "smoker's cough." Therefore the disease may be well advanced before a person seeks medical aid. Early diagnosis is of major importance for surgery or radiation therapy to be effective.

Obesity

An ever-growing problem in the United States is obesity, which, depending on its severity, produces alveolar hypoventilation and pulmonary restriction. This results from the thoracic contents being squashed up into the chest by an overdistended belly, which limits descent of the diaphragm. Such patients have a marked decrease in expiratory reserve volume and are more susceptible to postoperative respiratory complications.

The *Pickwickian syndrome,* a term used to describe a group of clinical features found in patients with extreme obesity, originates from a description by Charles Dickens of a fat boy. The term was applied by a group of investigators to their findings about obese patients (see chapter references). Clinical features of the Pickwickian syndrome are extreme obesity, somnolence, twitching, cyanosis, periodic respiration, polycythemia, right ventricular hypertrophy, and right ventricular failure. Arterial blood gas studies in these patients reflect alveolar hypoventilation with an increase in arterial P_{CO_2} and a decrease in arterial P_{O_2}.

Somnolence and fatigue are often symptoms that will bring the patient to the hospital. Patients will fall asleep sitting or even standing; it can occur in the middle of a conversation or some other light activity and will eventually become a source of embarrassment to the patient. The somnolence is caused by the elevation of arterial P_{CO_2} and hypoxemia. Dramatic weight reduction is the treatment for the Pickwickian syndrome, which results in a most impressive return of the patient's pulmonary function status to normal.

Obese patients present certain problems in terms of medical and nursing management, mainly because of their bulk. Hospital beds seem small, special tracheostomy tubes are required to traverse adipose tissue of the neck, and, most important, mobilization is difficult. Because of already reduced ventilatory function (which in turn increases the possibility of atelectasis), the obese patient requires vigorous respiratory care to prevent respiratory complications, and mobilization is absolutely essential.

REFERENCES

Ayres, S. M.: Beta receptors, cyclic AMP and the sympathetic nervous system, Respir. Care **17:**410-414, 1972.

Bates, D. V.: Air pollutants and the human lung, The James Waring Memorial Lecture, Am. Rev. Respir. Dis. **105:**1-13, 1972.

Cancer facts and figures, New York, 1976, The American Cancer Society.

Cherniack, R. M., Cherniak, L., and Naimark, A.: Respiration in health and disease, ed. 2, Philadelphia, 1972, W. B. Saunders Co.

Crofton, J., and Douglas, A.: Respiratory diseases, ed. 2, Oxford, 1975, Blackwell Scientific Publications, Ltd.

Hodgkin, J. E., et al.: Chronic obstructive airway diseases; current concepts in diagnosis and comprehensive care, J.A.M.A. **232:**1243-1260, 1975.

Lertzman, M. M., and Cherniack, R. M.: Rehabilitation of patients with chronic obstructive pulmonary disease, Am. Rev. Respir. Dis. **114:**1145-1166, 1976.

Ministry of Health Report on Public Health: Mortality and morbidity during London fog of December, 1952, London, 1954, Her Majesty's Stationery Office.

Petty, T. L., and Nett, L. M.: For those who live and breathe with emphysema and chronic bronchitis, Springfield, Ill., 1969, Charles C Thomas, Publishers.

Petty, T. L., and Hudson, L. D., editors: Fifteenth Aspen emphysema conference (reversible airway disease, formerly called asthma), Chest **63**(supp.):4, 1973.

Sobel, E.: Save your breath, a guide for people with chronic lung disease, Philadelphia, 1975, J. B. Lippincott Co.

The health consequences of smoking—a report of the Surgeon General, Pub. No. (HSM) 71-7513, Washington, D.C., U.S. Public Health Service, Department of Health, Education, and Welfare.

Wilson, A. F., and Galant, S. P.:, Recent advances in pathophysiology of asthma, West. J. Med. **120:**463-470, 1974.

7 / FOUNDATIONS OF RESPIRATORY CARE

Major advances in management of the patient with respiratory problems have occurred only within the last 20 years and many of these in the last decade. It is from these advances that the foundations of respiratory care have developed. The result is improved patient care and reduction in patient mortality from respiratory complications or disease.

This chapter is designed to present the nurse with the basic foundations of respiratory care, which include the intensive respiratory care unit and the respiratory intensive care team with their specific functions.

Because retention of secretions is a major respiratory complication, special emphasis has been placed in this chapter on early recognition and treatment of this complication through chest physical assessment, clinical interpretation of the chest x-ray film, and chest physiotherapy.

INTENSIVE RESPIRATORY CARE UNIT (IRCU)

Patients requiring intensive respiratory care should be nursed in an area equipped and staffed for that purpose. However, frequently other critical care areas and the medical and surgical wards are filled with patients who fall into this category. To deal with the problem many facilities assign four to six beds within an intensive care unit specially for patients in acute respiratory failure. These patients may have respiratory complications secondary to other conditions (automobile accidents, burns, drug ingestions, myocardial infarctions), or they may present with acute exacerbations of a chronic respiratory condition.

Physical set-up

Ideally a respiratory care unit should have single rooms built around a central nursing station. Each room should have a window (if possible) decked with bright, cheerful curtains. Sliding doors with the top section in glass add to the spaciousness of the room, allow the patient to be observed, and provide windows when a unit has none. The advantages of single rooms are that a patient (1) has privacy, (2) is not exposed to noise from ventilators or monitoring devices of other patients, (3) is not witness to the unpleasantness of emergency resuscitation on a fellow patient, and (4) is less exposed to cross-infection.

Whether or not a single room unit is possible, each bed in the respiratory care unit should be equipped with oxygen, compressed air, suction equipment, cardiac monitoring and defibrillation equipment, a clock, a calendar, and a bulletin board. The last three items are important to the psychologic aspects of respiratory nursing care.

Any architectural means of keeping equipment off the floor space around a patient's bed should be employed. This includes wall outlets for suction, oxygen, and compressed air; overhead intravenous poles; shelving for monitors; wall-bracketed blood pressure apparatus; and built-in cupboards to provide storage areas for material essential to patient care. The more clutter there is around a patient the easier it is for equipment to become disconnected and accidents to occur.

Special equipment

An intensive respiratory care unit must be equipped to cope with any cardiopulmonary emergency. Both volume-cycled and pressure-cycled ventilators should be available, as should instruments for gas analysis and instruments to measure simple tests of pulmonary function. (The cardiopulmonary emergency is discussed in Chapter 10.)

A mobile spirometer facilitates easy measurement of simple tests of pulmonary function such as vital capacity and rates of flow. In some facilities these are conducted daily by the nursing staff. Measurement of *end tidal carbon dioxide* levels (which are usually within 3 mm Hg of arterial carbon dioxide levels) by continuous infrared CO_2 analyzers provides an accurate method of intermittent monitoring of a patient's CO_2 level when no chronic lung disease exists. This is of value during long-term management of the respiratory patient when less frequent monitoring of arterial blood gases is desirable (for example, in a patient with a neuromuscular disorder whose blood gas results are fairly stable but, because of the possibility of further hypoventilation, a knowledge of the CO_2 level is desirable).

A number of Douglas bags, three-way valves, mouthpieces, adaptors for endotracheal and tracheostomy tubes, nose clips, and a stopwatch should be at hand for collection of expired gas samples. Important measurements of respiratory function can be obtained by this method (p. 193).

Oxygen analyzers and instruments for measuring expired gas volume should also be available. A close link between the pulmonary function laboratory and the respiratory care unit facilitates the use of equipment that is not normally available to critical care areas and saves duplication of expensive instruments.

Staffing

Intensive respiratory care requires that a patient be nursed continuously through each 24-hour period by highly skilled nursing staff. One nurse to each patient is ideal, and at least one nurse to two patients is essential for quality patient care and for safe nursing management. Patients undergoing intensive respiratory care, particularly those on mechanical ventilators, should not be left alone for one minute; therefore staff should be provided to relieve each nurse for meals and other breaks.

A relief-nurse system employed by the intensive care unit at Stanford University Hospital works effectively in the following way. A staff nurse working in the unit is assigned to "float" between three rooms during an entire shift. The responsibilities of the relief nurse include relieving the nurses in the assigned rooms for meals, assisting with nursing care (vital signs, turning, stripping chest tubes, etc.), replenishing stock supplies such as dressings and syringes, and assisting in emergency resuscitation. The relief nurses, in fact, do everything possible to assist their colleagues and to provide better patient care.

The advantage of such a system is that the unit is in a position to cope with a large number of severely ill patients. Nursing is done on a one-to-one or a one-to-two basis without a patient ever being left alone. It provides extra staff during emergencies so that (to an extent) other patients will not be deprived of intensive nursing care.

INTENSIVE RESPIRATORY CARE TEAM

Quality respiratory care emerges through the sustained efforts of a skilled medical team. Personnel assigned to such a team include a physician director, chest physicians, anesthesiologists, nurses, physiotherapists, respiratory therapists, and auxiliary personnel.

Physician members

Usually an intensive respiratory care unit will have a physician director who is responsible for leading the respiratory care team. Duties include establishing unit protocol and respiratory care standards, staff education, and direction of fellow physician members of the team. Physicians from the anesthesia service and respiratory service will generally participate as respiratory care team members.

Close liaison between respiratory care unit head nurses, instructors, supervisors, and the physician director is important in maintaining definitive rules as to what is within nursing practice and what is not. No gray area should exist, particularly with regard to crisis intervention; nurses should be completely aware of their boundaries.

Nursing staff

A nurse assigned to the intensive respiratory care unit, whether as a head nurse, a clinical specialist, an instructor, or a staff nurse, should be well trained in total patient care. These nurses should be proficient in nursing patients requiring ventilatory assistance, tracheostomy, controlled oxygen therapy, chest tubes, and cardiac monitoring. They must be able to recognize life-threatening situations, such as an obstructed airway or critical cardiac arrhythmia and be capable of crisis intervention.

Many facilities have large enough departments of physiotherapy and respiratory therapy to provide adequate service to the intensive respiratory care unit. This, however, should not give nurses a feeling of "that's their job" or "I don't need to know anything about that." Intensive respiratory care nurses are the medical personnel who are at the patient's bedside continuously, 24 hours a day, and they should become familiar with many aspects of respiratory therapy and physiotherapy in order to provide total patient care.

It is the responsibility of any nurse in a critical care area to keep up with current nursing concepts by reading journals for the profession. Respiratory care staff nurses should be provided with continuing on-the-job training and in-service education. This is conducted by physician members of the respiratory care team and nurse clinical specialists and/or instructors who have a working knowledge of pulmonary physiology and who are fully conversant with the many aspects of respiratory problems.

Intensive respiratory care nursing is demanding but also exciting and most rewarding. This stems in part from the wide variety of patients who need respiratory care and from the fact that good nursing care can mean the difference between recovery or further respiratory complications. Many facilities have already recognized the need for skilled nurses in this area and have established *pulmonary nurse* training programs to provide nurses with a background in pulmonary physiology and respiratory management.

Many universities are now offering master's degrees in pulmonary nursing, and pulmonary associates and specialists are being trained all over the United States.

Physiotherapists

The value of physiotherapists in the respiratory care team cannot be overemphasized. Through their daily routines of educating lazy muscles and instructing in various breathing techniques, physiotherapists develop a tremendous rapport with patients. I have seen these well-trained people aid in weaning the most frightened patients from respirators and in ambulating patients (after extensive therapy) who most medical personnel could not conceive would walk again.

The role of the physiotherapist in the respiratory care team is usually to provide extensive chest physiotherapy, which will prevent respiratory complications through the removal of pulmonary secretions and correct breathing techniques. Rehabilitation is also a service provided by the physiotherapy department and is most important in managing and training patients with chronic lung disease.

It should be remembered that many patients without a respiratory disease can develop respiratory failure. Whether these are patients with burns, trauma from automobile accidents, neuromuscular disease, or a postoperative complication, the physiotherapist works with the entire body not just the chest.

Nurses should learn as much as possible of the techniques of physiotherapy so that they are able to provide this aspect of patient care when such services are not available. Some of these techniques will be presented later in this chapter.

Respiratory therapists

Well-trained respiratory therapists are important members of the intensive respiratory care team. It is their responsibility to understand and operate the commonly used ventilators, to have an understanding of the effects of mechanical ventilation on the cardiopulmonary system, to provide routine respiratory therapy treatments for patients not on continuous ventilation, to be familiar with all forms of gas therapy, humidification, and nebulization, and to actively participate in cardiopulmonary resuscitation.

Many facilities do not have respiratory therapy services, and there is no reason why nurses cannot master any of the techniques just mentioned. Even when a large staff of respiratory therapists is available, it is not practical for them to handle the total respiratory care of a patient, such as suctioning, turning, and intermittent hyperinflation. They are not at the patient's bedside continuously; only the intensive respiratory care nurse is.

Auxiliary services

All hospital services are important to total patient management, and the valuable functions of the clinical laboratory, central sterile supply services, housekeeping, and so on should not be overlooked. Of the auxiliary services, some are specifically essential to effective functioning of the respiratory care team in patient management.

"Stat" laboratory. Whenever possible, a 24-hour laboratory service should be available to the intensive respiratory care unit. Such a service must have the highest standards of quality control because patient management often depends on the results obtained. The importance of prompt, accurate laboratory information on the critically ill has led some facilities to develop the "stat" laboratory. In one such laboratory, within 11 minutes of receiving a sample of blood twenty-three measurements are made and reported back to the unit. Blood gas results are available in 3 to 5 minutes.

Arterial blood gas measurements are most important to the critically ill patient because, depending on the test results, respirator settings may be changed, a patient may be intubated, sodium bicarbonate may be administered, or a patient may be "weaned" from the respirator.

ASSESSMENT OF THE RESPIRATORY PATIENT

One of the most important aspects of respiratory nursing care is clinical observation—look at and listen to the patient. An example of the significance of this aspect of care was well demonstrated during a seminar I attended. A speaker had delivered an excellent lecture on computerized monitoring. On the blackboard were a list of the advantages of such a system. When the next speaker came to the podium to discuss the recognition of postoperative respiratory complications, we noticed written across the blackboard in large red letters, "A well-trained nurse." The speaker then proceeded to explain how to use the wonderful gifts of our own vital senses, which we so often overlook in this technologic age.

Our assessment skills not only involve use of particular vital senses (seeing, hearing, touching, and smelling) but the application of medical knowledge to these senses. For example, looking at a patient informs us of the patient's approximate age, sex, obvious emotional distress, body size and shape, skin texture and color (cyanosis or pallor), presence of digital "clubbing," body deformity, use of accessory muscles of respiration, labored breathing, excursions of the chest, position of the trachea, and the presence of edema.

Sensory data once received can be then interpreted, used with our existing knowledge, and acted on to set priorities and make decisions.

When assessing the respiratory patient, a medical history is obtained and a physical examination is conducted, paying particular attention to examination of the chest.

Obtaining a history

To obtain accurate information from a person, it is essential to open the doors of communication between both parties. Many psychologists have attempted to help us master skills that will enable us to talk with people more honestly and freely and to guide others into talking with them in the same way. Dr. Thomas Gordon is a psychologist who has devoted much time to helping people communicate through "Effectiveness Training." His techniques in "Nurse Effectiveness Training" courses are designed to help nurses communicate better with patients and colleagues.

Two of Dr. Gordon's fundamental techniques are what he calls "door openers" to communication and "passive listening." Simple door openers to communication are presented here.

"I see."

"Really?"

"Is that so?"

"Interesting."

"Tell me more about it."

"I'd like to hear about it."

"Sounds like you've got something to say about this."

"This seems like something important to you."

"Let's hear what you have to say."

Passive listening is a silent listening process based on a genuine and wholehearted desire to hear what the patient has to say. These techniques can be most useful when obtaining a history from a patient. They allow the patient to do most of the talking.

Introduction. When first meeting the patient, it is important to say who you are, why you are there, and who sent you. However gentle and kind your approach may be to a patient, he may still view you as one of those persons in the medical profession who is just bursting with knowledge—so very much more than he has. It is therefore essential to try to establish a common ground of early conversation, a warm ground. Pick something at the patient's bedside: a book, a photograph, anything that makes you feel comfortable making an introduction on a more personal level. Try to avoid direct interrogation. "Is that a picture of your grandson?" sounds personal, but the photograph may be of his son, which would probably make you both feel uncom-

TABLE 4. Checklist for history taking of the pulmonary patient

Chief complaint	Order of collecting data
General findings	Chief complaint
Fever	Present illness
Weight loss	Family history
Anorexia, nausea, vomiting	Respiratory history
Fatigue	Social history
Sleep patterns	Occupational history
Exercise tolerance	Environmental factors
Pulmonary findings	Review of systems
Postnasal drip	Physical examination
Cough	Laboratory data
Sputum production	
Amount	
Color	
Hemoptysis	
Chest pain	
Dyspnea	
Wheezing	
Digital clubbing	

fortable. Also, questioning is already so much a part of his hospital stay that he may well be tired of it. Another approach might be, "My, what a handsome boy in the photograph." This gives the patient a chance to respond in his own way.

Collecting the information. All data should be collected in an orderly fashion. Table 4 provides a *checklist* for taking a simple history from a pulmonary patient. When using the checklist, it is important to present the material in terms of *onset* and *duration:* When did it begin? How long has it been going on?

The next step elaborates on the checklist by putting those findings in terms of the *present illness.* This is accomplished using the following method:

1. *Body location.* Where is the symptom located?
2. *Quality.* What is it like?
3. *Quantity.* How intense is it?
4. *Chronology.* When did the symptom begin and what course has it followed?
5. *Setting.* Under what circumstances did it occur?
6. *Aggravating and alleviating factors.* What makes it worse or better?
7. *Associated manifestations.* What other symptoms or phenomena are associated with it?

When time is a limiting factor (as in the critical care setting), I have found it best to go through the checklist, collect information on the present illness, and conduct the physical examination. The additional information can be collected at another time.

Physical examination of the chest

When examining the chest, the nurse should look for abnormalities in structure and function that may be caused by respiratory diseases and for complications. The techniques used to conduct a chest physical examination are inspection, palpation, percussion, and auscultation. These should be carried out in a well-lighted room in relative peace and quiet whenever practical.

Inspection. To inspect the chest adequately the patient should be stripped to the waist. A female patient will need a folded hand towel to cover her breasts during certain portions of the examination of the anterior chest. Have the patient in a sitting position when possible to get a total look at the chest. Note the skin color and look for any skin lesions or abnormalities, such as the spider nevi seen in cirrhosis of the liver, or scars, which may indicate previous thoracic surgery. Look for any structural alterations in the thorax, such as deformity (for example, kyphoscoliosis), or an increase in the anteroposterior diameter of the chest, which may indicate chronic obstructive airways disease. As you continue to look at the patient, notice (and count) the rate and depth of breathing and whether it is of a regular, rhythmic quality or whether it is irregular, labored, or sighing, indicative of distress. Also, when observing the quality of respiration, it is important to note the ratio of inspiration to expiration, which is normally 1:2. In chronic obstructive disease, expiration is usually prolonged. Notice the position in which the patient chooses to breathe. Is the pose typical of the patient with emphysema: leaning forward with hands on his knees or with arms folded on the bed table? Look to see whether the patient is using accessory muscles of respiration to help him to breathe, a sign associated with chronic obstructive pulmonary disease. Also observe for uniformity in chest expansion. Nonuniformity occurs when one side of the chest cannot expand to the same degree as the other. This is seen in pneumothorax, obstruction of a major bronchus, fractured ribs, or guarding due to pain.

Inspiratory retraction of the interspaces should also be looked for. This may be due to fibrosis of the underlying lung or emphysema. In a severe asthma attack, retraction will be marked. Bulging of the intercostal spaces indicates loss of thoracic structure such as occurs with several fractured ribs.

Palpation. Frequently inspection and palpation are carried out simultaneously. This allows a hands-on check to what the nurse sees and also provides additional data. For example, to confirm symmetry (the uniformity of chest expansion), place your hands lightly on both sides of the anterior chest so that the thumbs touch the sternal border. If the chest moves uniformly during inspiration, your thumbs will separate equal distance.

The nurse palpates the chest to look for chest wall tenderness or masses, enlargement of cervical, supraclavicular, and axillary lymph nodes, and to note the position of the trachea. The chest is also palpated for the vibrations transmitted to the chest wall during speech, termed *vocal fremitus;* when these vibrations are palpated, the term is *tactile fremitus.* Tests for tactile fremitus are done by having the patient repeat words such as "ninety-nine" or "one-two-three," maintaining the same pitch and intensity of voice each time. At the same time the examiner places the *palmar* base of the fingers against the apices of the posterior chest and compares the vibrations felt (with the same hand) from one side of the chest to the other, moving down the chest to the lung bases. The procedure is then repeated over lateral and anterior aspects of the chest.

Tactile fremitus normally varies in intensity with voice pitch: high-pitched voices produce poorer vibrations than do low-pitched voices. For this reason women may have to be asked to use a lower voice than normal during the procedure. Intensity of tactile fremitus is normally much greater over the parasternal region, which corresponds with major bronchial bifurcation. It is also greater in the intrascapular region. In disease an increase in vocal femitus occurs where there is increased transmission of sounds, such as in consolidation from pneumonia or a lung abscess. Vocal femitus is less palpable or may be absent when there is dampening to the transmission of sound as in pleural effusion, pneumothorax, or pleural thickening.

Percussion. Of the techniques in chest physical examination, percussion probably requires the most practice. If you have attempted this portion of the examination on a sick patient and think you have heard nothing that could be interpreted, it is best to wait rather than try again. Practice whenever possible on healthy volunteers or unconscious patients. Sick patients really do not appreciate the second thumping.

To percuss the chest, press the palmar surface of the middle finger of one hand *lightly* into an interspace in the area of lung to be percussed, then strike it sharply (on the distal knuckle) with the tip of the finger on the other hand, using a swinging movement. This movement has been compared with the head of the woodpecker as it strikes a tree. During percussion the sounds of each side of the chest are compared with the same area on the opposite side.

Certain percussion notes are listened for as the procedure is carried out. Normally the air-filled lung has a resonant percussion note. A hyperresonant note occurs when there is an increase in the amount of air in the lung as with pulmonary emphysema.

In pathologic conditions when there is a decrease in the amount of air present in sections, there is a decreased resonance, spoken of in terms of flat percussion notes and dull percussion notes. A dull percussion note is elicited when the heart is percussed and when there is consolidation or atelectasis present in the lung.

Auscultation. The act of listening to sounds in various parts of the body with a stethoscope is known as auscultation. Before attempting to listen to a patient's chest, make sure that your stethoscope has no leaks in it, that the earpieces fit snugly in your ears, and that the diaphragm is warmed a little. An easy check that the stethoscope is functioning is to gently tap the diaphragm while the earpieces are in your ears.

Auscultation of the chest with a stethoscope is performed in a bilateral fashion from left to right, with the nurse listening to corresponding areas of the patient's chest. Thus corresponding areas on either side can be compared. The diaphragm of the stethoscope is pressed firmly against the patient's skin.

Breath sounds. As air travels through the airways, sounds are transmitted that are called breath sounds. There are normal and abnormal breath sounds. They are heard during inspiration and expiration, with particular attention given to the length of each phase of respiration. The longer the phase the louder will be the sound in that phase.

Vesicular breath sounds are normal and are heard as a whishing sound over all but the largest airways in the lung. They are characterized by a smooth progression from inspiration to expiration, with inspiration being longer than expiration. Vesicular sounds are heard as a result of the movement of air in the alveoli; they are soft sounds, with the expiratory phase being quite faint.

Bronchovesicular sounds can be *normal* or *abnormal*. These sounds are normally present at the level of the manubrium sterni (closest to the main stem bronchi) in the second to third interspace. They are of a more hollow tubular quality, and expiration is longer and thus louder than inspiration. The sound occurs as air travels through larger airways and the major bronchi.

Tracheal sounds also have a loud tubular quality and are normally heard over the trachea. Tracheal breathing closely resembles the abnormal bronchial breath sounds.

Bronchial breath sounds are abnormal, have a relatively short inspiratory phase, a long expiratory phase, and an audible gap between inspiration and expiration. Bronchial sounds have a blowing, whooshing quality to them and are generally heard in conditions that facilitate the transmission of sound in the bronchial tree such as occurs with consolidation.

Bronchovesicular breath sounds also occur in pathologic conditions of the lung that cause consolidation or compression of the normal lung. In lung disease, bronchovesicular sounds are heard in areas of the lung other than over the large airways.

Adventitious sounds. There are four main types of adventitious sounds: rhonchi, rales, wheezes, and pleural friction rubs. Adventitious means added extrinsically, not innate; therefore adventitious sounds are *always abnormal* and occur with pathologic changes in the lungs and tracheobronchial tree.

Rhonchi may be thought of as dry sounds that are musical in quality. They are heard generally during expiration but occasionally during inspiration. *Rhonchus* comes from the Latin word meaning to wheeze, which gives a clue to the type of condition and where the sounds come from. Rhonchi are associated with diseases of the airways such as asthma, in which the changes in airway caliber affect the way air flows through them. When rhonchi are heard during expiration only, it means that there is still a little elasticity to the airway allowing the airway to open and air to pass through during inspiration. If rhonchi are heard during inspiration and expiration, they suggest that total spasm of the airway is present.

Rhonchi are frequently extensive in the asthmatic patient just after a bout of exercise or just before medication is due. They may frequently be produced in the bronchitic or asthmatic patient by having the patient forcibly exhale at speed. Rhonchi may also be heard following suctioning for removal of secretions.

Rales are moist sounds, nonmusical in nature, and are usually divided into three categories: (1) fine, also known as crepitant; (2) medium; and (3) coarse. Rales are usually heard late in the inspiratory phase of respiration, and they occur with alveolar and interstitial diseases such as pneumonia, pulmonary edema, purulent bronchitis, or pulmonary fibrosis.

Crepitant rales are produced by moisture in the alveoli and small airways and are usually heard in the periphery of the lung. Patchy atelectatic areas may produce fine rales, which may disappear after the patient has coughed or following chest physiotherapy. A sound like a rale, which comes from the French word for rattle, may be closely duplicated by rubbing a thin strand of hair between the thumb and forefinger close to the ear. Rubbing of the skin or hair with the diaphragm of the stethoscope also produces a sound like rales.

Medium rales are heard over medium airways (lobar bronchi). Coarse rales occur both with inspiration and expiration, giving them a continuous quality. The sound is bubbling, caused by moisture in the larger airways, such as large amounts of secretions. It is frequently heard in the patient who requires suctioning and may disappear if the secretions are cleared.

Sometimes coarse rales are termed rhonchi. I believe that there is less confusion if rales and rhonchi are separated into wet and dry sounds which can occur in the same patient at the same time.

Wheezes are musical in quality, heard as a high-pitched whistling sound mainly during expiration. Wheezing occurs with airway narrowing and is heard in patients with asthma.

During a recent asthma research project, I had the opportunity to auscultate the chests of the participants over an 8-hour period. On many occasions it was really rather like listening to a full symphony tuning up prior to performance.

Pleural friction rubs are loud grating sounds heard with inflammation of the pleura as the two surfaces rub together. The sound is heard over an extremely limited area during the latter part of inspiration and also on expiration. This sound may be duplicated by rubbing a finger over an inflated balloon.

Diffuse interstitial fibrosis causes a unique sound that can be heard close to the surface of the chest wall and is like the sound of Velcro fastenings as they are pulled apart.

The finding that breath sounds are *absent* or *diminished* is an indication that there is no movement of air in that particular area of lung. This may have occurred as a result of atelectasis or where there is collapse of a lobe or segment due to blockage of the airways leading to that portion of lung. Routine hourly auscultation of the critically ill patient will alert the nurse to these kinds of changes as well as the development of adventitious sounds.

Voice sounds. When words are spoken, vibrations are set up and transmitted through the bronchial tree. Patients are usually given test words like "ninety-nine" to say and then the chest is auscultated to hear the sounds transmitted. Sometimes the test words are said in a whisper. Normally the transmission of the sound will be faint, and during auscultation the whispered syllables will not be distinct. The term *whispered pectoriloquy* is used when test words said in a whisper are heard as loud sounds.

Whispered pectoriloquy is extremely useful in early detection of pneumonia and atelectasis. Under these circumstances the whispered test syllables are heard clearly and distinctly with the stethoscope. This sign is termed *bronchophony*. *Egophony* is the term used when the "E" sound spoken by a patient comes out as an "A" sound, or when the syllables have a peculiar nasal bleating quality. This may be caused by pleural effusion and the compressed lung beneath it or also with consolidation.

When auscultating the chest for breath sounds, it is important to obtain the best quality by having the patient breathe in and out through his open mouth slowly and deeply. Some sounds, such as rales, may disappear after coughing. Thus the patient should be asked to cough. Note whether a spasm of the airways heard as rhonchi can be induced by having the patient perform a forceful exhalation: take a deep breath in then blow out as hard and fast as possible.

HUMIDIFICATION AND NEBULIZATION

Normally during inspiration, ambient air is satisfactorily warmed and humidified as it passes through the conducting airways so that at body temperature alveolar air is 100% saturated with water vapor (Chapter 2). Conditioning of inspired air is important to mucus production, ciliary activity, and a healthy respiratory tract. When normal function is interfered with, other methods of adding moisture to the respiratory system must be undertaken. These methods are referred to as humidification and nebulization. The latter method also serves as a delivery route for certain medications.

Humidification

Adequate humidification is an absolute necessity in preventing respiratory complications and is indicated as follows: (1) whenever a dry gas is administered to a patient, (2) when the nasopharynx is bypassed by endotracheal intubation or tracheostomy, (3) in the presence of thick, tenacious secretions, and (4) in the relief of croup or tracheitis.

Oxygen is a dry gas (STPD) as it is delivered from its supply source, and moisture *must* be added to it prior to its administration to a patient. The moisture added is usually water, which should be in a sufficient quantity to saturate the gas with water vapor at a body temperature of 37° C.

Normally 75% of humidification takes place in the nasopharynx. This is eliminated when a patient is treated by endotracheal intubation or tracheostomy. Therefore adequate humidification of the inspired air is vital to these patients.

Nebulization

A second method of adding moisture to the inspired air is by the addition of water droplets of varying sizes. This is accomplished through the process of nebulization. When fine solid or liquid particles are in suspension in a gas, this is known as an aerosol, and most nebulizers are designed to deliver a maximum number of particles of the desired size. Thus the nebulizer delivers aerosol therapy through nebulization, and the term *aerosol* is commonly used in the place of, or interchangeably with, *nebulization.*

Liquid or solid particles are of various sizes and range from less than 0.1 micron up to 50 to 60 microns in diameter. Particles of less than 0.1 micron enter the respiratory tract and are deposited by the process of diffusion at the alveolar level. Particles of 1 to 3 microns reach the smaller bronchioles, and particles of 50 to 60 microns are deposited in the upper airway and the tubes of the delivery system. It is desirable, therefore, when using nebulization as a means of adding water to the respiratory tract, to use equipment that will deliver extremely fine water particles. Clinical indications for the use of nebulization are the same as those for humidification. Medications such as bronchodilators are, however, more commonly administered by a nebulizer.

There are many types of equipment available for humidification and nebulization, some of which overlap in function. They may have heating elements or work at room temperature. A commonly used method of humidification of an inspired gas is a bubble-diffusion humidifier, which adds water vapor to the gas in an amount determined by temperature and bubble size. This is accomplished as the gas passes through a tube with a porous head, which is immersed in a water bottle. Some units, such as the cascade humidifier that is used with a mechanical ventilator, work on the principle of the bubble-diffusion humidifier but have the added advantage of a heating element, which allows a gas to reach the patient 100% saturated with water vapor.

A jet-aerosol humidifier or jet nebulizer requires the use of gas under pressure. The simple hand-bulb nebulizer works on this principle; a gas enters the fluid chamber through a narrow opening and a mist is created. This type of equipment is often used in conjunction with a heating element for oxygen or mist therapy with compressed air.

The ultrasonic nebulizer produces the finest water particles. It works on the principle of high-frequency vibrations which, through a complex system, are transmitted to break up water into fine particles. These particles are carried from the nebulizer and are efficiently deposited throughout the tracheobronchial tree. Ultrasonic nebulization has proved to be most effective clinically in the liquefaction of thick or inspissated secretions that occur in conditions such as obstructive pulmonary disease (especially cystic fibrosis). Although efficient, the ultrasonic nebulizer may also cause complications by delivering too much water to the patient, causing excessive secretions and exacerbation of bronchospasm.

CHEST PHYSIOTHERAPY

One major complication arising in sick, immobile patients is the collection of pulmonary secretions, which may predispose atelectasis or pneumonia. This is a particular danger during the early postoperative period for any patient and is a serious problem in the aged. In patients with lung disease such complications are further compounded by the underlying respiratory disorder. It is with these points in mind that the basic objectives of chest physiotherapy are formulated: (1) *prevention* of respiratory complications, (2) *correction* of such complications where possible, and (3) *improvement* in pulmonary function.

Prevention of respiratory complications

In surgical patients a preoperative chest physiotherapy program, which is continued in the postoperative period, is of great value in preventing respiratory complications. During the preoperative period, patients should be taught correct breathing and coughing techniques and should be provided with information regarding the effects of the surgical procedure on their respiratory function. This is best accomplished by the trained physiotherapist who will be caring for the patient during the preoperative and postoperative periods.

An essential ingredient in such a program is the rapport that therapists establish with their patients. From this point a therapist will go on to give a full explanation of the aims of the physiotherapy program, placing particular emphasis on the importance of relaxation as a means of preventing muscle tension and pain. Patients are usually made aware of the excursions and expansion of their chest wall during inspiration and expiration and are taught full use of their respiratory muscles.

In preventing postoperative respiratory complications, good nursing care incorporates three simple principles of chest physiotherapy—*turn, deep breathe,* and *cough.* These are familiar basic nursing principles, which should be implemented during the immediate postoperative period and continued until the patient is able to move around freely. Every member of the nursing team should be aware of the importance of those four small words and see that they are incorporated as standard nursing procedure even when a patient cannot be moved. For example, even the patient who has undergone delicate eye surgery can do deep breathing exercises, which are essential for hyperinflation of alveoli and prevention of respiratory complications.

Studies have shown that when the normal sigh (which occurs about eleven times each hour) is suppressed by anesthetic agents or drugs, the incidence of atelectasis increases. Periodic hyperinflation, which a sigh provides, is believed to inflate those alveoli that are not inflated during tidal breathing and to be involved in surfactant production.

Turning. Immobile patients must be turned. This may appear to be impossible, for example, in a patient who has been in a motorcycle accident and has multiple fractures. The solution in a situation like this may be the addition of a spiker bar between the two lower limb casts, which will allow balanced and easy turning of such patients. This example is presented to emphasize that all possibilities must be explored before deciding that it is *impossible* to turn even the most awkward of cases.

A side-back-side-back-side routine is used where possible to turn patients. In the immediate postoperative period side-side positioning is more desirable until the patient has recovered completely from anesthesia. Thus the chances of aspiration or blockage of the airway by the tongue are reduced. The number of times that a patient is turned during a 24-hour period varies with his condition and a physician's orders. Certain other techniques of chest physiotherapy that utilize position are essential in intensive respiratory care and will be discussed later in this section.

Deep breathing. Pain is one of the most important limiting factors to deep breathing. When this results from surgical trauma to the thorax or abdomen, movement of the chest wall is also limited and tidal volume is reduced. This combination can easily result in respiratory complications, unless good breathing habits are encouraged. Most effective are deep breaths, which are taken slowly, deliberately, and to full chest expansion. I find patients will do much better when I place my hands (warmed first) on one or both sides of the lower rib cage so that they can feel chest expansion taking place. Doing the exercise with the patient always helps.

If surgical patients take in a breath too quickly, chances are that they will have pain from the effects of sudden changes in intrapulmonary pressure on the thorax or abdomen, which will make them afraid of deep-breathing exercises. Therefore nurses must give much support and encouragement to these patients.

Cough. One most important natural mechanism for the removal of secretions is coughing. A cough is usually a reflex mechanism stimulated by irritation of the respiratory tract by secretions or foreign material such as smoke or inhalation of fluid or food particles by accident. A cough is performed by taking a deep breath, closing the glottis, and forcefully contracting the muscles of expiration (particularly the abdominal muscles). As intrapulmonic pressure increases, the vocal chords separate, and as the entrapped air is rapidly expelled, secretions are dislodged and expectorated. In patients in respiratory failure the normal cough is often suppressed by drugs or may be limited because of pain or because the glottis has been bypassed with endo-tracheal intubation or tracheostomy. Coughing is an important protective mechanism for the lungs, and every effort must be made to overcome these limited factors and to encourage effective cough.

Trauma to the chest wall or abdomen from either a surgical incision or accidental injury will initially prevent a patient from coughing because of the pain encountered. Much pain can be alleviated if (1) vigorous chest physiotherapy is coordinated after the administration of an analgesic, (2) the patient's wound is stabilized by the nurse or therapist during coughing, and (3) correct deep breathing and coughing techniques are taught to the patient.

Correction of respiratory complications

Respiratory complications can occur despite good nursing care and preventive chest physiotherapy. In some patients the complications were present when they were admitted (for example, the patient who aspirates vomitus following ingestion of large amounts of a drug, the drowning victim, or the patient with severe lung disease). Chest physiotherapy to correct respiratory complications involves the removal of two types of pulmonary secretions—macrosecretions and microsecretions.

Macrosecretions are those pulmonary secretions found in the large bronchial tubes and are removed by coughing, suctioning, postural drainage techniques, and percussion. *Microsecretions* are those secretions found in smaller bronchial tubes and bronchioles and are *not* easily removed. They cannot be reached by suctioning, and postural drainage techniques have little effect in their clearance. Some of the chest physiotherapy techniques used to deal with pulmonary secretions are postural drain-age, percussion, and vibration.

Postural drainage. A traditional technique employed in chest physiotherapy is postural drainage, or "tipping," whereby pulmonary secretions can be drained by gravity from the segments of each lung into major bronchi and are then removed by coughing or suctioning. As the name implies, patients are postured; that is, they are

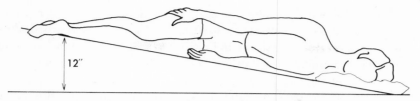

FIG. 7-1. Alternate position for middle-lobe drainage.

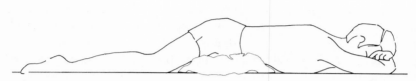

FIG. 7-2. Position for lower-lobe drainage, apical segments. Raising the foot of the bed 18 inches with the patient in this position will also drain the posterior basal segments.

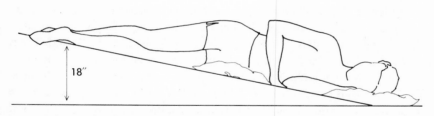

FIG. 7-3. Position for lower-lobe drainage, lateral basal segments.

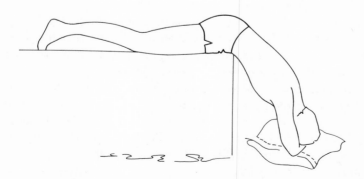

FIG. 7-4. Jackknife position for lower-lobe drainage, posterior basal segments.

placed in various positions to attain drainage. Although other positions can be used in postural drainage, those that can be used most effectively at the bedside even when a patient is severely ill are shown in Figs. 7-1 to 7-4. Most of these positions can be incorporated into routine turning of patients, except for the dramatic tipping illustrated in Fig. 7-4.

Equipment required when postural drainage is conducted includes tissues, a sputum cup, and extra pillows. If the patient is undergoing mechanical ventilation, suction equipment will, of course, be at the bedside. The procedure is explained to the patient, making sure that the treatment does not immediately precede or follow a meal. Any tight clothing or binders are loosened and the patient is encouraged to deep breathe and cough prior to positioning and between position changes. If the patient has chest x rays routinely, the radiologist's report should be checked to find out which lobe will require the most drainage. When physicians order chest physiotherapy for a patient they will usually indicate the area of lung requiring the most vigorous treatment.

The most common areas of lung for secretions to collect are the lower and middle lobes.

Drainage of secretions from the *middle lobe* on the right side or the *lingular lobe* on the left side is performed by positioning the patient on his side, with his head downward (if tolerated) about 30 degrees. This is done by raising the foot of the bed 12 inches. A pillow is placed behind the patient's shoulder and hip and he is gently rolled back onto them, with the uppermost arm behind the hip. The area over the nipple (not in female patients) and under the axilla is then percussed and vibrated. The patient is encouraged to deep-breathe and cough, and then is positioned the same way on the opposite side. Another technique for middle-lobe drainage, which will also drain medial, anterior, and certain basal segments of the lower lobes, is illustrated in Fig. 7-1. The patient is positioned on his side with the uppermost shoulder thrown slightly forward; body balance is maintained by positioning the upper leg behind the lower. This is a comfortable position and is easily incorporated in nursing care.

The *lower lobes* are drained by segment, and the position shown in Fig. 7-2 illustrates the position for drainage of the *apical segments*. Percussion and vibration are done over the scapula. Drainage of the *posterior basal segments* of the lower lobes is accomplished using an exaggeration of the same position by raising the foot of the bed 18 inches. Percussion and vibration are then carried out over the lower ribs. The *anterior basal segments* are drained by placing the patient on his back in the Trendelenburg position with a pillow under his knees and raising the foot of the bed 18 inches. Percussion and vibration are performed over the lower ribs. In the latter positions it is important to protect the patient's head from the headboard or bedrail by adequate padding or shoulder supports. *Lateral basal segments* of the lower lobes are drained with the patient positioned on his side, head downward, knees slightly bent, and the foot of the bed raised 18 inches (Fig. 7-3). Percussion and vibration are performed over the exposed lower rib cage.

The most effective position for draining the posterior basal segments of the lower

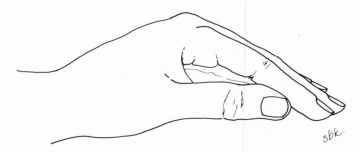

FIG. 7-5. Cupped hand position for percussion.

lobes is not tolerated by seriously ill patients, and the modified version just described is more suitable in many instances. When the exaggerated position can be used, the patient is positioned keeping his back as straight as possible and draping the whole trunk over the end of a high bed or tilt-table to assume a jackknife position (Fig. 7-4). The patient folds his arms and places them on a pillow on the floor in front of him, thus providing support for his head and trunk. Many patients, particularly those with chronic bronchitis or cystic fibrosis, use the jackknife position at home two or three times a day to clear secretions.

After postural drainage a patient should be given mouth care and placed in a comfortable position. The quantity and character of the expectorated or suctioned secretions should be observed and charted. A fresh sputum container should be used so that it can be weighed before and after treatment. A small household scale is a valuable piece of equipment for this purpose.

Percussion. To aid in dislodging pulmonary secretions, the physiotherapy technique of manual percussion is employed. Terms such as *clapping* and *tapping* may be used and mean the same thing. Both hands are generally used in alternating, uniform, rhythmic percussion of the chest over the lobe where secretions have collected. Best results are accomplished with the nurse's hands in a slightly cupped position (Fig. 7-5), which will create an air pocket between the hand and chest wall and allow a more forceful maneuver. A hollow sound, not a slapping sound, should be heard. To avoid tiring the arms, the wrists must be entirely loose and the elbow slightly flexed. This technique is performed during or following postural drainage. It requires only 2 to 3 minutes and is a most valuable part of the physiotherapy routine. Although a technique of force, the patient should not experience pain during percussion and any tender area should be avoided. If properly performed, the patient will find this technique soothing, and muscular relaxation with sputum expectoration will follow.

Vibration. While postural drainage and percussion may not be effective in removal of *microsecretions*, vibration of the chest often will dislodge the most stubborn secretions in both large and small airways. This technique is aimed at literally shaking loose secretions and is best accomplished by placing the hands (arms and shoulders straight) on the patient's chest at the level of secretions and then applying pressure, followed by continual vibration for about 10 seconds. Chest vibration is more effective when conducted during a slow, forceful expiration.

The three techniques presented—tipping (postural drainage), percussion, and vibration (TPV)—are chest physiotherapy techniques that are conducted as combined therapy at one time. A patient is positioned and tipped for 10 to 15 minutes, then percussion, vibration, and removal of secretions are followed by coughing or suctioning, before turning the patient and placing him in the next position. TPV may be ordered half-hourly, hourly, every 2 hours or every 4 hours. A half-hourly chest physiotherapy program of anything more than turn, cough, and deep breathe is most demanding on patients and staff alike and is not suitable. An hourly program may be necessary when a patient has excessive secretions and is not on mechanical ventilation. However, the 2-hourly program is probably the most desirable for most patients.

BASIC INTERPRETATION IN CHEST ROENTGENOLOGY

When assessing patients, it is important not only to look at the physical findings but also at all other available data. This includes looking at the chest roentgenogram, or chest x-ray film as it is usually called. In critical care settings, chest x-ray films are frequently taken to assess changes in lung pathology, to check for correct placement of an endotracheal tube, or to look for the presence of pleural fluid or pneumothorax. A nurse at the bedside can soon learn to recognize these conditions in the chest film once the basic steps to interpretation have been mastered.

What is an x-ray film? The x-ray process in medicine began when Wilhelm Roentgen (1845-1923) discovered that cathode rays used in a certain way would emit x-rays that were of a wavelike form similar to light. The importance of this type of wave variety is that it has the ability to penetrate relatively opaque substance. X-rays belong in the electromagnetic spectrum along with visible light rays, infrared, etc. When x-rays come in contact with photographic film, a chemical reaction is set up, and the exposed film is black.

When the x-ray beam enters a person, some of the rays pass directly through the patient. This shows as the black areas. Some rays are absorbed by thoracic structures before reaching the film, and some are scattered. The different degree to which the thoracic structures (heart, mediastinum, lymphatics, ribs) absorb x-rays causes the photographic shadows seen on a chest film.

Chest x-ray densities. When chest x-ray films are interpreted, the degrees of blackness on the film are compared either with each other or against a film taken earlier. There are four types of densities (blackness) seen on a chest film. These are *gas* or *air*, *water*, *fat*, and *metal* (Table 5). Gas is the least dense and therefore absorbs minimal x-rays; thus air-filled structures such as the lungs appear the blackest on the film. Water density is seen with soft tissue, muscle, and blood. The heart appears as water density, which is lighter than gas density. Even lighter is fat density, and the lightest of all is metal density seen in bony structures such as the ribs because these absorb the most rays.

Water density is an important factor in interpreting chest films. For example, the
Text continued on p. 117.

TABLE 5. Normal x-ray densities seen in a chest film

Gas	Water	Fat	Metal
Lungs Trachea Bronchi Alveoli	Heart Muscle Blood Aortic knob Aorta Diaphragm Vessels	Some streaking of fat in the hilar region	Ribs Clavicles Scapulae Vertebrae

TABLE 6. Types of chest x-ray films that may be ordered

Type of film	Position of patient	X-ray tube position
Posteroanterior (PA)	Upright	Horizontal at 6 feet from film
Anteroposterior (AP)	Supine or sitting in bed	Vertical if supine; horizontal if sitting; as close to 6 feet from film as possible
Left lateral	Upright, both hands above head with film held against left side	Horizontal with beam directed at right side of chest
Right lateral	Upright, both hands above head with film held against right side	Horizontal with beam directed at left side of chest
Left or right decubitus	Lying down on left or right side	Horizontal; tube faces left or right side at 6 feet from film
Lordotic	Upright	At angle of 45 degrees, 6 feet from film

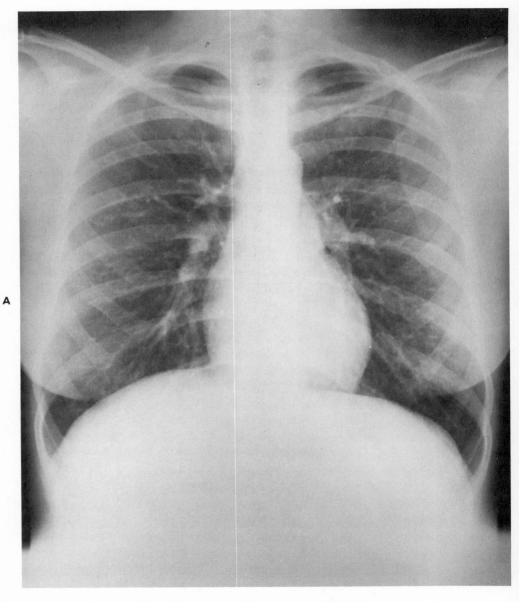

FIG. 7-6. A, Normal posteroanterior chest film.

Right

Left

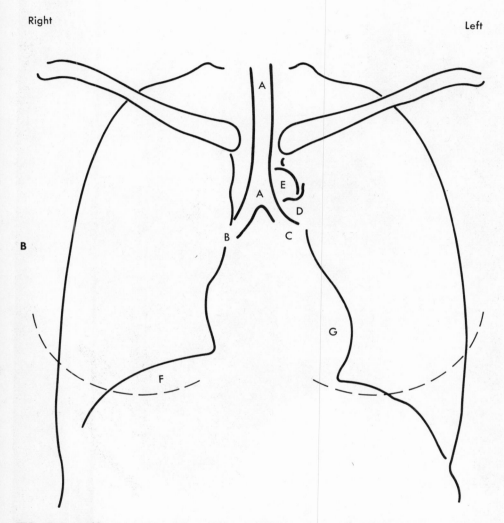

FIG. 7-6, cont'd. B, Outlines of anatomic structure that correspond to posteroanterior chest film, **A.** *A,* Trachea; *B,* right main stem bronchus; *C,* left main stem bronchus; *D,* position of left pulmonary artery; *E,* aortic knob; *F,* right hemidiaphragm; *G,* left heart border. Broken lines indicate breast shadows seen in female patients.   *Continued.*

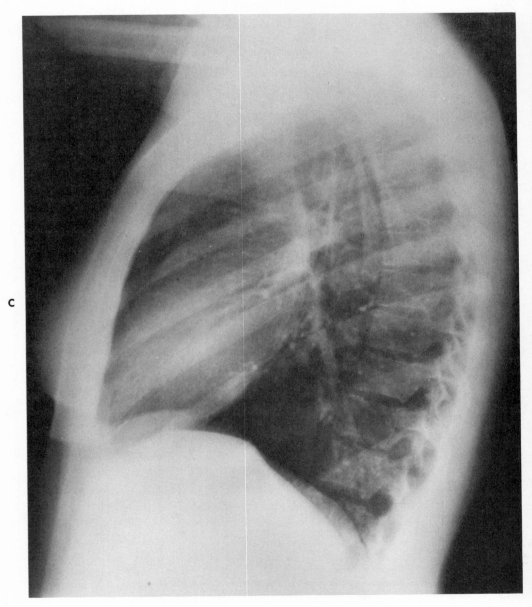

FIG. 7-6, cont'd. C, Normal right lateral chest film.

heart and great vessels comprise three water densities: blood, muscle, and the soft tissue of the vessels. Yet they are all seen as one. Thus, if a disease state converts the air-filled lung to a fluid-filled lung (water density), the area involved may obliterate or deform the existing outline of the heart or any other water-density structure with which it makes anatomic contact.

Types of chest x-ray films. There are many types of chest x-ray films that can be ordered (Table 6), but those most commonly seen are the posteroanterior (PA), anteroposterior (AP), and the left or right lateral. These terms refer to the direction in which the x-ray beam passes through the patient, for example, from back (posterior) to front (anterior) in the posteroanterior film.

The distance away from the patient at which the film is taken is important to the degree of magnification and sharpness of the film. It is ideal to have a film that shows images with extreme sharpness and the least magnification. An adequate chest film is obtained at a distance of approximately 6 feet from the patient's chest.

The type of chest film that is most commonly taken in critical care settings is the anteroposterior (AP) view, in which the x-ray beams pass from front to back. The equipment for this is frequently portable. The quality of a portable chest film is somewhat inferior to that of the film taken in the x-ray department because of incorrect positioning of the patient and the difficulty of placing the x-ray machine 6 feet away from the patient. To reduce these factors the patient should be sitting completely upright or standing at the bedside if at all possible with the x-ray machine the correct distance away. Lead aprons should be worn by personnel in the area when the film is being taken to protect against the scattering of x-rays.

A normal chest film is usually taken during inspiration. A film taken on exhalation will look a little cloudy, and the cardiac silhouette may be larger, which can lead to interpretation of pathologic changes that do not exist.

There are uses for an expiratory film, however; these include pneumothorax, where the condition may be missed under certain circumstances during inspiration; and with pulmonary emphysema, where there is air retained at the end of exhalation.

Interpretation of the chest film. What are nurses actually looking at and looking for when interpreting the chest film? First, the film is placed on the viewing box so that, when the nurse faces the film, the right side of the chest will be on the nurse's left and the left side of the chest on the right. The left side is usually easily identified because the major portion of the heart lies on that side. Second, knowing the types of densities, the nurse can now identify various structures (Fig. 7-6). There are also certain signs to be looked for in the presence of cardiopulmonary disease that will be examined here.

The *silhouette sign* is seen when a border of the heart, aorta, or diaphragm comes into anatomic contact with a condition producing water density and is obliterated by it. In the normal chest film there is no silhouette sign. The anatomic contact of the lobes of the lung and their relationship to the heart and aorta provide the landmarks for locating the disease process. For example, a right middle lobe pneumonia would show loss of the silhouette of a major part of the right heart border because the greater portion of this border is in contact with the anterior segment of the right middle lobe.

The *air bronchogram sign* is seen when a disease process allows the nurse to observe the bronchi as intrapulmonary black tubular structures. Normally bronchi are not seen because they are air-filled structures (gas density) surrounded by other air-filled structures, the alveoli. Once the lung tissue around the bronchi changes to water density with disease, then the air-filled bronchi can be seen. Disease processes such as pneumonia, pulmonary edema, pulmonary infarcts, and bronchiectasis can produce an air bronchogram sign.

The significance of an air bronchogram sign is that only diseased tissue containing bronchi can produce it, which pinpoints the disease location outside of the mediastinum, chest wall, or pleura, since these areas do not contain bronchi.

Many conditions lead to *collapse* of a lobe segment or whole lung, which may be seen on the chest film. The three major causes of collapse are *obstruction, compression,* and *contraction.* Obstructive collapse is spoken of in terms of being central, peripheral, intrinsic, or extrinsic. For example, if an obstruction is central, a bronchus is blocked by a single process such as a foreign body (intrinsic) or by pressure from enlarged lymph nodes (extrinsic). When the obstruction is peripheral, it is caused by several bronchi being plugged with mucus or exudate. Atelectasis is an example of peripheral obstruction. Obstructive collapse occurs because the air distal to the blockage is absorbed by the pulmonary capillary blood flow, and the lobe or segment collapses.

Pneumothorax is an example of collapse by compression. As the air enters the pleural space, the higher atmospheric pressure is exerted on the lung and forces the air out, and the lung collapses. A pleural effusion may also cause compression collapse as the fluid exerts pressure on the lung and forces air out.

Disease entities that bring about contraction collapse are pulmonary fibrosis, radiation pneumonitis, asbestosis, and silicosis.

The whole lung or a collapsed portion of it appears as increased blackness on the chest film with free air seen as much darker gas density. Air-filled bullae from pulmonary emphysema may have a similar appearance.

The chest films shown in Figs. 7-7 and 7-8 illustrate two case histories.

References on p. 124.

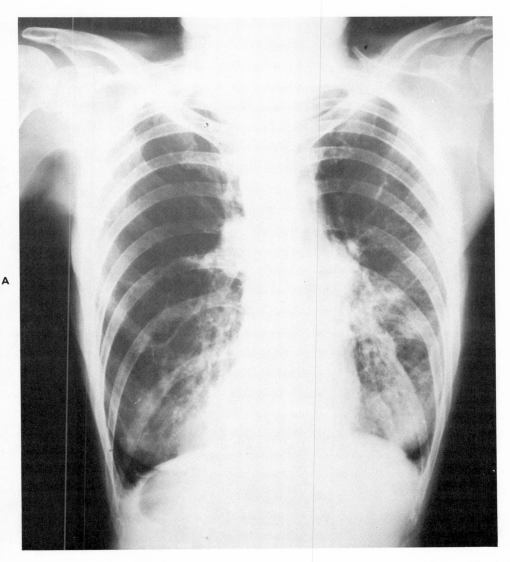

FIG. 7-7. A, A 69-year-old female with a history of chronic obstructive pulmonary disease was admitted with dyspnea. The initial chest film at 3:00 AM, **A,** shows a small left pneumothorax, which has caused a shift of the heart and mediastinum to the right. (When collapse of an entire lobe or a lung occurs, the mediastinal structures will most frequently be seen to shift to the affected side rather than away from it.) When comparing this with the normal chest film (Fig. 7-6), it can be seen that the heart borders are not clearly defined (silhouette sign) because of patchy infiltrates from pneumonia. *Continued.*

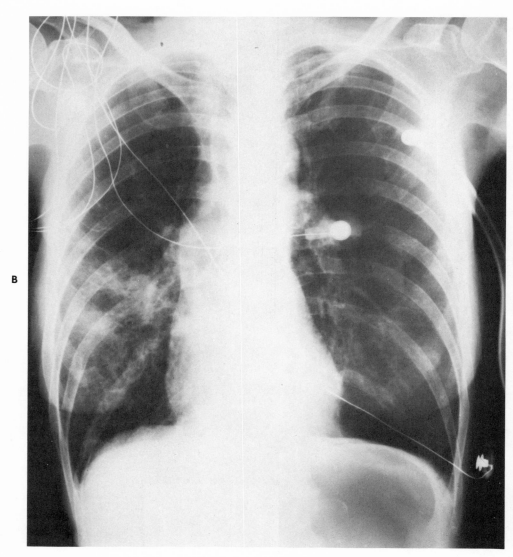

FIG. 7-7, cont'd. A second chest film was obtained, **B,** following insertion of a chest tube (visible in the left upper lobe) and some reexpansion of the left upper lobe. This is seen as a fine black line of separation between the collapsed and expanded portions of lung. The heart and mediastinum have returned to the midline, and the outline of the left heart border is more clearly defined. Note that there is some clearing of the pneumonia in the right lower lobe. There is some gastric distention seen by the large air bubble under the left hemidiaphragm. Electroencephalogram leads are also visible.

FIG. 7-7, cont'd. A film taken the next day, **C,** shows the chest tube still in situ but also an increase of pulmonary infiltrates, mainly on the right side. These are due to pneumonia, which is an example of peripheral obstructive collapse.

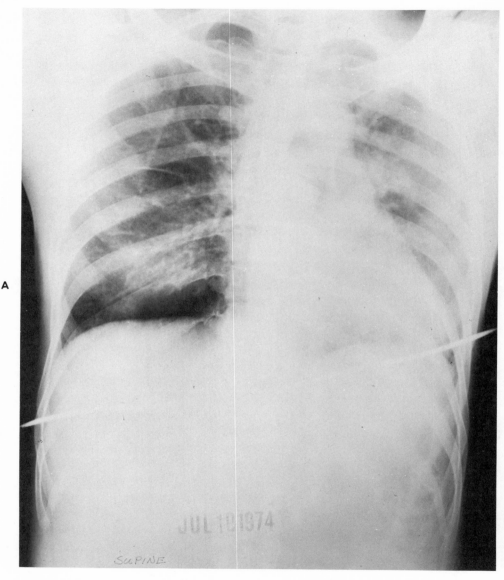

FIG. 7-8. A, A 37-year-old male, undergoing mechanical ventilation by way of an endotracheal tube, had diminished breath sounds on the left side of the chest. **A** is a portable supine anteroposterior film which shows that the endotracheal tube is positioned in the right main stem bronchus. The tube lines can be followed down the trachea slightly to the left-hand side. There is partial collapse of the left lung, with a shift of the heart and mediastinum toward the left due to atelectasis. The tube was repositioned and, with adequate ventilation and physiotherapy, repeat films (not shown) suggested significant improvement in the patient's condition.

FIG. 7-8, cont'd. This anteroposterior film, **B,** taken of the same patient the next day, after weaning from mechanical ventilation and extubation, shows reexpansion of the left lung and clear lung fields. A normal chest film.

REFERENCES

Broughton, J.: Chest physical diagnosis for nurses and respiratory therapists, Heart Lung 1:200-207, 1972.

Felson, B., Weinstein, A. S., and Spitz, H. B.: Principles of chest roentgenology, Philadelphia, 1965, W. B. Saunders Co.

Fowkes, W. C., and Hunn, V. K.: Clinical assessment for the nurse practitioner, St. Louis, 1973, The C. V. Mosby Co.

Fuhs, M., Rieser, M., and Brisbon, D.: Nursing in a respiratory intensive care unit, Chest 62(supp.): 14-18, 1972.

Gold, M. I.: The respiratory care unit, Heart Lung 1(3):378-383, 1972.

Michaels, S.: The stat laboratory (abstract), 14th Annual Symposium on Critical Care Medicine, San Francisco, 1976.

Petty, T. L., and Farrington, J. F.: The intensive respiratory care unit, Clin. Notes Respir. Dis. 10:3-11, 1971.

Physiotherapy for medical and surgical thoracic conditions, London, 1967, Physiotherapy Department, Brompton Hospital.

Schooley, E.: An introduction to x-rays of the cardiopulmonary system (learning module), Baltimore, 1976, The Williams & Wilkins Co.

Sitzman, J.: Nursing management of the acutely ill respiratory patient, Heart Lung 1:207-213, 1972.

Sykes, M. K., McNicol, M. W., and Campbell, E. J. M.: Respiratory failure, Oxford, 1969, Blackwell Scientific Publications, Ltd.

Tinker, J.: Understanding chest x-rays Am. J. Nurs. 76:54-59, 1976.

Winslow, E. H.: Visual inspection of the patient with cardiopulmonary disease, Heart Lung 4:421-429, 1975.

8 / HYPOXEMIA, HYPOXIA, AND OXYGEN THERAPY

Advances in bedside monitoring techniques now provide enough data to assess a patient's cardiopulmonary status accurately in terms of oxygen uptake consumption and delivery. These advances, however, have also made it necessary to have a complete understanding of the physiologic principles behind the collection of such sophisticated data. Chapters 1 through 5 have described much of the detailed physiologic aspects of respiratory care. Now these can be expanded and applied to the serious conditions of hypoxemia and hypoxia and their treatment with oxygen therapy.

HYPOXEMIA AND HYPOXIA

You will recall that hypoxemia is a reduction in the level of oxygen in arterial blood (oxygen tension) and that hypoxia is a reduction in the amount of oxygen delivered to the tissues to meet metabolic needs of the body. Some of the possible causes of hypoxia are listed in Table 7. When looking at the table you will note that the four major causes of hypoxemia are listed as causes of hypoxia, which indicates that hypoxemia results in hypoxia. The four major causes of hypoxemia are (1) ventilation-perfusion abnormalities, (2) alveolar hypoventilation, (3) venous-arterial shunts, and (4) diffusion defects. These were briefly discussed in Chapter 5, but because of their clinical importance will be presented in more depth. A list of the conditions that result in each of these causes is presented in Table 8.

Ventilation-perfusion abnormalities. Abnormalities in distribution of alveolar ventilation with respect to blood flow are common to cardiopulmonary disorders and are a major cause of hypoxemia. As previously stated, distribution of alveolar ventilation ($\dot{V}_A$) and blood flow ($\dot{Q}$) is uneven in the normal upright lung. This is due to gravity and changes in hydrostatic and transmural pressures up the lung. There is, however, a mean value for the ratio of alveolar ventilation to blood flow of 0.8. This figure is arrived at by taking the ratio of normal alveolar ventilation of approximately 4 liters/min to pulmonary blood flow of 5 liters/min ($\dot{V}_A$ liters/min : $\dot{Q}$ 5 liters/min = 0.8). The term *ventilation-perfusion relationships* is used interchangeably with $\dot{V}_A/\dot{Q}$ *relationships*.

An *increase* in ventilation-perfusion ratio indicates that there is too much ventilation in relation to blood flowing through the area. Thus some alveolar ventilation is wasted and contributes to the alveolar dead space and hence the physiologic dead

TABLE 7. Possible causes of hypoxia

Predisposing factor	Possible cause
Reduction in inspired oxygen concentration	Altitude Faulty equipment
Reduction in arterial P_{O_2}	$\dot{V}_A/\dot{Q}$ abnormalities Hypoventilation Shunts Diffusion defects
Reduction in oxygen-carrying capacity of blood	Anemia Abnormal hemoglobin Carbon monoxide poisoning
Reduction in cardiac output	Myocardial infarction Decreased coronary perfusion Cardiac arrhythmias Increased vascular resistance
Increased oxygen requirement	Extreme obesity Fever Burns

TABLE 8. Causes of hypoxemia

Ventilation-perfusion abnormalities	Alveolar hypoventilation

Regional ventilation abnormalities
   Pulmonary emphysema
   Bronchial asthma
   Chronic bronchitis
   Carcinoma
 Regional perfusion abnormalities
   Pulmonary embolus
   Pulmonary infarction
   Decreased cardiac output
	Interference with respiratory center activity
	   Drugs
	   Central nervous system disturbances
	 Restriction to lung and/or alveolar expansion
	   Emphysema
	   Pulmonary fibrosis
	   Pneumothorax
	   Pleural effusion
	 Reduced thoracic expansion
	   Surgical trauma
	   Pain
	   Fatigue
	   Deformity
	 Obesity

Venous-arterial shunts	**Diffusion defects**
Atelectasis Pneumonia Shock Fluid overload Pulmonary emboli Pulmonary edema Prolonged oxygen therapy	Pulmonary edema Sarcoidosis Radiation pneumonitis Destruction of pulmonary capillary bed

space (Chapter 4). For example, when an embolus blocks a large pulmonary vessel, there will be little or no blood flow to some ventilated alveoli to add carbon dioxide to the *alveolar gas* or to remove oxygen. In response to the increased carbon dioxide level, overall ventilation will increase, which will maintain the arterial PCO_2 within normal limits, but the reduction in the alveolar PCO_2 will persist because there is no change in the alveolar dead space. The increase in ventilation has little effect on the arterial PO_2, and hypoxemia is present. Measurement of the difference between arterial and mixed expired alveolar carbon dioxide tension will be reflected as a widening (gradient) because of the reduction in carbon dioxide added to the alveolar gas. This situation results only in increases in ventilation relative to perfusion.

Other perfusion abnormalities that increase the $\dot{V}_A/\dot{Q}$ ratio are a reduction in cardiac output and pulmonary vasoconstriction, which leave some normally ventilated alveoli poorly perfused. Again blood that has a reduced oxygen tension will be added to the arterial blood.

A *decrease* in the ventilation-perfusion ratio occurs when there is maldistribution of ventilation with respect to blood flow. The result is venous admixture because the blood passing by the poorly ventilated alveoli is not fully oxygenated. This occurs in conditions such as asthma, in which airway narrowing limits normal distribution of ventilation or emphysematous changes to alveolar structure.

The conditions that most commonly cause $\dot{V}_A/\dot{Q}$ abnormalities are presented in Table 8. At a glance many of these appear to be those listed as a cause of hypoventilation. The difference is that in $\dot{V}_A/\dot{Q}$ relationships *regional distribution* of ventilation with respect to blood flow is the key factor, and unlike abnormalities that cause hypoventilation, this distribution is not usually associated with elevated carbon dioxide levels.

The hypoxemia caused by $\dot{V}_A/\dot{Q}$ abnormalities is relieved when oxygen is administered to the patient.

Alveolar hypoventilation. When a patient is breathing room air, alveolar hypoventilation always results in hypoxemia and hypercapnia. The causes of alveolar hypoventilation are presented in Table 8. The relationship between alveolar ventilation and the levels of carbon dioxide in arterial blood is almost linear. Thus if alveolar ventilation is halved, carbon dioxide is doubled.

When oxygen is administered to the patient with alveolar hypoventilation, the hypoxemia will be relieved; however, this will do nothing to restore adequate ventilation and thus will not remove the excess carbon dioxide.

Venous-arterial shunts. In respiratory medicine the type of shunt that is spoken of is the *physiologic shunt*, which means that a percentage of blood has not come into contact with ventilated alveoli and is therefore never exposed to alveolar oxygen; this results in venous admixture.

In the normal lung a small amount of venous blood bypasses the ventilated lung and mixes with arterial blood, resulting in a shunt. This shunted blood comes in part from the bronchial venous blood of the systemic circulation and in part out of the Thebesian veins from the myocardium, which drain into the left heart. From 1% to 2% of the cardiac output constitutes the normal physiologic shunt and causes a decrease in arterial Po_2 of about 5 mm Hg in a person breathing room air.

In the critically ill patient high percentages of venous blood are shunted to the arterial side because frequently large areas of lung will be atelectatic, congested, or obstructed with a large proportion of alveolar collapse.

Although physiologic shunts and $\dot{V}a/\dot{Q}$ abnormalities cause venous admixture, the hypoxemia from $\dot{V}a/\dot{Q}$ abnormalities will disappear with oxygen administration, but the hypoxemia caused by shunting will not. To determine the difference between a low ventilation-perfusion ratio and blood that never comes into contact with ventilated alveoli, the patient is given 100% oxygen to breathe over a 20-minute period by way of a closed system using a nose clip. With a low ventilation-perfusion ratio eventually all the nitrogen will be washed out of the alveoli and the arterial blood will reach full oxygenation regardless of how poorly ventilated certain alveoli are with respect to blood flow. This will be reflected by an arterial Po_2 of 580 to 600 mm Hg when the patient receives 100% oxygen. However, if venous blood is never exposed to alveolar oxygen, breathing 100% oxygen will not raise the patient's arterial Po_2 to the desired amount.

Diffusion defects. The fourth cause of hypoxemia is a defect in the normal rate of gas transfer across the alveolar-capillary membranes. Conditions that cause diffusion defects involve conditions that alter the size of the diffusion pathway or alter the structure of the alveolar-capillary bed.

Pulmonary edema widens the diffusion pathway, and the rate of gas transfer is reduced because of the presence of interstitial and intra-alveolar fluid. In conditions such as sarcoidosis, radiation pneumonitis, and interstitial fibrosis, the alveolar wall becomes thickened and less permeable to gases.

Destruction of portions of the pulmonary capillary bed resulting from pulmonary emboli will also affect the rate of gas transfer. Diffusion defects are frequently *not* considered as an important cause of hypoxemia because the conditions involved could also be thought of in terms of ventilation-perfusion abnormalities. However, a pure diffusion defect will cause a reduction in the diffusion capacity of the lung (Chapter 4), whereas patients with $\dot{V}a/\dot{Q}$ abnormalities usually will have no reduction in their diffusion capacity.

Disease processes that cause hypoxemia frequently occur concurrently with other conditions that result in hypoxia, particularly in the critically ill patient. For example, patients in intensive care units often incur a large venous-arterial shunt due to atelectasis, may be anemic, have cardiac arrhythmias, and may be febrile. Each condition leads to more hypoxia. *Hypoxia* is a complex condition that may result from imbalances in oxygen uptake, transport, delivery, or utilization by tissue cells. Let us examine each of these more closely.

Inadequate oxygen uptake. For oxygen uptake to be adequate there must be a normal fractional concentration of oxygen in the inspired air (Fi_{O_2}), which must reach the alveoli through normal ventilation. Alveolar oxygen molecules must then be able to diffuse across the alveolar capillary membranes, where adequate perfusion with blood containing a normal hemoglobin will pick up the oxygen molecules. The causes of hypoxemia presented earlier will all affect oxygen uptake as will a reduction in the inspired oxygen concentration.

The factors that predispose a reduction in FI_{O_2} are either faulty equipment used in the delivery of oxygen or a lower ambient pressure as occurs at altitude.

The normal barometric pressure at sea level is 760 mm Hg, whereas in Denver, Colorado, the barometric pressure is 625 mm Hg. However, the FI_{O_2} when an individual is breathing room air is still 20.94%; thus the partial pressure of inspired air, PI_{O_2}, will be reduced.

$$PI_{O_2} = \frac{20.94 \times (625 \text{ mm Hg} - 47 \text{ mm Hg})}{100} = 121 \text{ mm Hg}$$

Altitude adjustment for persons with normal lungs brings about little alteration in function. One of the advantages of the oxyhemoglobin dissociation curve is that a small reduction in inspired oxygen will not greatly affect the arterial oxygen saturation.

Inadequate oxygen transport. Oxygen transport is dependent on normal functioning of the cardiovascular system, the concentration of hemoglobin in the blood, the affinity of hemoglobin for oxygen, the inspired oxygen concentration, and tissue metabolism.

A major impairment in cardiovascular function is a *reduction in cardiac output*, which will reduce the amount of blood flow throughout the circulation and hence the amount of blood flow to the tissues. In response to a fall in the amount of blood flow, the tissues will *extract* more oxygen from the blood available to meet their metabolic requirements. This, in turn, reduces the saturation of the venous blood returning to the heart.

A way of determining tissue oxygen extraction is to measure the difference between the oxygen saturation of arterial blood (Sa_{O_2}) and that of mixed venous blood (Sv_{O_2}). A sample of arterial blood has a saturation of 95% to 97%, and a sample of mixed venous blood taken from the pulmonary artery or the right ventricle has a saturation of 70% to 75%. The difference of 20% to 25% is representative of normal tissue oxygen extraction at rest.

Another guide to the efficiency of oxygen transport and uptake is to measure the arteriovenous (a-v) oxygen difference. This is accomplished by deducting the oxygen content of mixed venous blood (15 vol%) from the oxygen content of arterial blood (20 vol%), which usually yields a difference of 5 vol%. This value reflects arteriovenous oxygen difference for the body as a whole and does not show the difference from organ to organ. For example, the heart, which is a highly metabolic organ, has an a-v oxygen difference of about 11.4 vol% compared with the skin's 1 vol%.

Changes in the normal concentration of hemoglobin, such as in anemia or polycythemia, results in altered oxygen transport. You will recall that oxygen is carried by hemoglobin as oxyhemoglobin. Therefore a reduction in hemoglobin concentration as a result of hemorrhage or anemia from any cause can reduce the amount of oxygen transported in the blood to the tissues.

The regulation of red blood cell production is believed to be governed by tissue oxygenation and the production of a glycoprotein called *erythropoietin.* Production of erythropoietin is thought to occur as a result of renal hypoxia. In the presence of hypoxia an enzyme is released by the kidneys known as the renal erythropoietic stimulating factor. With the aid of this factor, erythropoietin is produced in the blood, where it is transported to act on the bone marrow to produce more red blood cells. It is known that in response to a decrease in oxygen transport to the tissues there is an increase in red blood cell production. The polycythemia seen particularly in patients with chronic hypoxia that occurs with pulmonary emphysema or as a result of high altitude adjustment is an example of this mechanism.

The affinity of hemoglobin for oxygen is also an important factor in oxygen transport. A *decrease* in the affinity of hemoglobin for oxygen corresponds with a shift of the oxyhemoglobin dissociation curve to the right and thus an increase in oxygen release to the tissues (Chapter 5).

Normal values for the affinity of hemoglobin for oxygen are expressed in terms of the oxygen tension necessary to saturate hemoglobin 50% at pH 7.40 and a body temperature of 37° C. This is known as the P_{50}, and looking at Fig. 8-1 one can see at a PO_2 of 26.6 mm Hg, hemoglobin is 50% saturated with oxygen. An increase in P_{50} may result from an increase in temperature, arterial carbon dioxide, hydrogen ion concentration (decreased pH), or an increase in blood levels of 2,3-diphosphoglycerate (DPG) or adenosine triphosphate (ATP).

As levels of DPG rise in the blood in response, for example, to hypoxia, the result is an increase in the value of P_{50} and, hence, the oxygen available to the tissues. Disease processes that cause an *increase in P_{50}* include shock, anemia, cirrhosis, congestive heart failure, chronic obstructive pulmonary disease, and hemoglobinopathies.

Decreased levels of DPG cause a decrease in the P_{50} value and a decrease in oxygen release from hemoglobin (an increased affinity). A decrease in P_{50} is also caused by carbon monoxide poisoning.

Signs and symptoms of hypoxemia and hypoxia. When looking for the signs and symptoms of hypoxia, we should recall that central and peripheral chemoreceptors in the body are sensitive to changes in levels of carbon dioxide and oxygen in the blood and that the peripheral chemoreceptors (the carotid and aortic bodies) are particularly sensitive to reductions in arterial PO_2.

The onset of hypoxia is mainly heralded by *subtle* changes in a patient's condition unless the cause is an obstructed airway or circulatory failure. Laboratory measurement of arterial PO_2 will easily reveal the degree of hypoxemia present, but the degree of hypoxia is less easily determined and can vary from organ to organ and cell to cell, depending on their oxygen supply, metabolic activity, and oxygen requirement.

The heart and the brain are both organs with high arteriovenous oxygen differences (extraction rate), and although the brain has some oxygen reserve, the heart has none. In response to hypoxia the body tries to compensate by increasing oxygen transport, which is manifested by an increase in ventilation, increase in cardiac output, and cerebral and coronary vasodilatation (in an effort to supply more blood to the brain and heart).

Altered cerebral function, manifested by restlessness, headache, irritability, or euphoria, may occur early with hypoxia and can progress with the degree of cerebral hypoxia present to delirium and coma.

Tachypnea may be the initial sign of an increase in ventilation, which may be felt as dyspnea by the patient.

Tachycardia may be the first indication of the increase in cardiac output and may be accompanied by hypertension. Hypertension occurs secondarily to increased cardiac output because of increased peripheral vascular resistance.

Definite clinical manifestations of hypoxemia and hypoxia, such as *central* or *peripheral cyanosis,* may not be observed until oxygen saturation has fallen to almost 78% or if the patient is anemic, which means that the arterial Po_2 is slightly above venous levels. If cyanosis is present from whatever cause, it is a clear indication for oxygen therapy.

In the critical care setting early detection of hypoxia on the basis of signs and symptoms may be difficult. Often with the use of drugs or in the presence of disease, normal compensatory mechanisms may be unable to function. One example of this is the patient with chronic lung disease who has a carotid endarterectomy and thereby loses his hypoxic response for stimulation of respiration because of damage to or loss of the carotid bodies. Another example is the patient in cardiac failure who cannot respond to hypoxia by increasing heart rate and thus cardiac output.

Cardiac output may also be compromised in hypoxia because of an increase in pulmonary vascular resistance, which means that there is increased work for the right side of the heart to pump the blood through the pulmonary circulation (Chapter 4). In hypoxia, although there is cerebral and coronary vasodilatation, there is pulmonary vasoconstriction, which accounts for the increase in pulmonary vascular resistance.

OXYGEN THERAPY

Thus far you have learned the way oxygen is taken up and transported by way of the blood and the many disturbances that can disrupt this mechanism.

This section will deal with the uses of oxygen therapy, the dangers of such therapy, clinical indications, and the methods of administration.

Uses of oxygen therapy

Oxygen therapy is used to *relieve hypoxemia* and *avoid hypoxia,* particularly of the heart and brain. Oxygen is not a substitute for other forms of treatment and should be used only when indicated. It should be borne in mind that oxygen is a *drug;* it has dangerous side effects and is expensive. The respiratory care team should be fully aware of such side effects and be able to recognize their clinical manifestations. Like any drug the dosage (concentration) of oxygen should be carefully controlled. It should be given in sufficient amounts to maintain an adequate arterial Po_2, which will vary from patient to patient.

Oxygen therapy without assisted ventilation does nothing to improve alveolar ventilation. It does, however, raise the inspired oxygen concentration and hence the alveolar oxygen level. This will be effective to a degree in relieving hypoxia from any of the causes listed in Table 7.

Dangers of oxygen therapy

Oxygen is an odorless, colorless gas that exerts a partial pressure of 150 mm Hg in atmospheric air at sea level. As previously stated, oxygen is a drug and should be thought of as such. In certain situations it is a dangerous drug and can result in severe lung damage and death. There are two main dangers of oxygen therapy—the physical dangers and the physiologic dangers.

Physical dangers. Although oxygen itself is not a flammable gas, it has properties that support combustion. No-smoking rules in hospital rooms must be enforced in the presence of oxygen therapy. By far the best way of accomplishing this is to have a hospital policy of no smoking in any patient area.

In places where high concentrations of oxygen are used under pressures greater than atmospheric (for example, in hyperbaric oxygen therapy), any spark may cause a fire. Extreme precautions must be taken under these conditions.

Physiologic dangers. A journal of physiology in London in 1899 published a paper written by Dr. J. Lorrain-Smith entitled "The Pathological Effects Due to Increase of Oxygen Tension in the Air Breathed." From this the Lorrain-Smith effect became known, which is the damage to the pulmonary epithelium found to occur following prolonged inhalation of high concentrations (over 60%) of oxygen. Although this physiologic danger was known so long ago, only recent studies have supported the Lorrain-Smith effect. High concentrations of oxygen administered over a period of time are now believed to damage alveolar epithelial cells and also inactivate production of pulmonary surfactant.

Atelectasis also occurs following administration of high concentrations of oxygen. This results from the effects of the nitrogen (normally 80% in the lungs) being washed out from the alveoli by the high concentration of oxygen. This complication is common in the well-sedated postoperative patient who has a low tidal volume and has a tendency to retain secretions. If alveoli are not hyperinflated by the natural sigh and become difficult to inflate because of the increase in surface tension (decreased surfactant), the result will be collapse.

Retrolental fibroplasia, which was once a major cause of blindness in infants who had been treated in the neonatal period with high concentrations of oxygen, is still a potential complication of oxygen therapy. It is now known, however, that the level of oxygen in the blood flowing to the retina is the important factor in controlling the condition. Most of the infants who require oxygen therapy in the neonatal period are those suffering from the respiratory distress syndrome, or hyaline membrane disease, and high concentrations of oxygen are often needed for them to achieve a normal arterial PO_2. Apparently if the arterial PO_2 is maintained within normal limits, there is little contraindication to high oxygen concentrations under these circumstances and no complications of blindness from retrolental fibroplasia are observed.

Oxygen-induced carbon dioxide narcosis is the best known physiologic danger of oxygen therapy. It is still a common complication encountered in clinical practice. This occurs in patients with chronic pulmonary disease who have chronic alveolar hypoventilation, and therefore chronic CO_2 retention and hypoxemia. Carbon dioxide is the most powerful stimulus to breathing, and a sudden rise in arterial PCO_2 will result in an immediate response by the respiratory centers to increase ventilation and thus eliminate CO_2. In these patients, however, the continuously high levels of PCO_2 (55 mm Hg and above) result in interference with the normal control of respiration. A sudden further rise in arterial PCO_2 for these patients results in complete inhibition in the respiratory center's response to CO_2, and the stimulus or drive to respiration becomes hypoxic. If oxygen is given to such patients under any except the most controlled conditions, hypoxic drive is removed, hypoventilation increases, CO_2 increases, and the patient will rapidly relapse into unconsciousness.

Oxygen toxicity is best thought of as the truly poisonous effect of the drug on the whole body. Some complications such as lung damage and atelectasis may be predisposing factors in oxygen toxicity. Other signs and symptoms are also indicative of toxicity.

Retrosternal pain has been found to occur in patients after 6 hours of receiving 100% oxygen at atmospheric pressure. The same symptoms occurred at 36 hours when the inspired oxygen concentration was 60%. If 100% oxygen is inhaled for 60 hours or more, it produces a rapid and continuous reduction in vital capacity. These effects appear to be most profound when oxygen administration is by mechanical ventilation. Several animal studies have revealed that death can occur from severe pulmonary complications within 2 to 10 days of continuous administration of 100% oxygen.

Acute poisoning of the central nervous system, resulting in convulsions, is known to occur particularly when oxygen is administered at pressures higher than 1 atm.

Although the complications of oxygen therapy are thought to be on the decline in these days of respiratory enlightenment, they will continue to be with us until everyone realizes and respects the potential dangers of increases in oxygen tension in the air breathed—as Dr. J. Lorrain-Smith did in 1899.

Clinical indications for oxygen therapy

Oxygen, despite its many dangers, is a highly valuable drug. Oxygen is necessary for life processes to continue, and it is essential in the relief of hypoxemia and hypoxia. Table 9 provides a list of common clinical indications for oxygen therapy, suggests the physiologic responses to those conditions, and presents a guide to the type of therapy used.

Controlled oxygen therapy

The principles and techniques of controlled oxygen therapy were developed in 1960 by Dr. E. J. M. Campbell, a physician who has contributed a great deal to all aspects of respiratory care.

Controlled oxygen therapy is designed for the patient with a chronic elevation of arterial PCO_2, abnormal respiratory control, and hypoxemia. If high concentrations

TABLE 9. Common indications for oxygen therapy

Condition	Arterial blood gases and physiology	Oxygen therapy

Decreased PI_{O_2}
  Faulty equipment
  Faulty O_2 administration
  Altitude
	Low PO_2 due to decreased PI_{O_2}; low CO_2 due to respiratory compensation of hyperventilation	Concentration to restore PI_{O_2} to normal

Chronic obstructive pulmonary disease with acute exacerbation	Low PO_2, high PCO_2 from alveolar hypoventilation and abnormal ventilation/blood flow relationships, hypoxic respiratory drive	Controlled oxygen therapy (see text) (*Never* use high concentrations of O_2.)

Respiratory depression
  Drugs
  Anesthesia
  Neuromuscular disease
	Low PO_2, high PCO_2 from alveolar hypoventilation; hypoxic respiratory drive	Mechanical ventilation with oxygen (*Never* use high concentrations of O_2 alone.)

Decreased cardiac output
  Myocardial infarction
  Cardiac arrhythmias
  Increased pulmonary vascular resistance
  Cardiogenic shock
	Low PO_2, variable PCO_2; abnormal ventilation/blood flow relationships and decreased regional blood flow	Higher concentrations of oxygen needed to relieve tissue hypoxia and restore PO_2

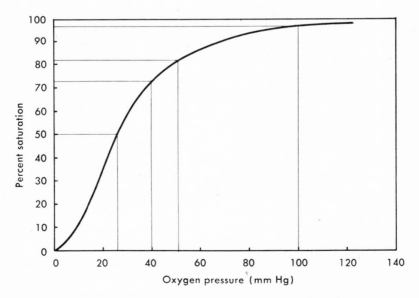

FIG. 8-1. Significance of increases in oxygen partial pressure and their effect on oxygen saturation. Note that when the partial pressure of oxygen is raised from 25 to 50 mm Hg, the saturation is increased over 30%. Also note that at a PO_2 of 26.6 mm Hg the saturation of hemoglobin is 50% (P_{50}).

of oxygen are given to such patients, there is a further elevation of P_{CO_2} and carbon dioxide narcosis. Yet the hypoxemia, which is often severe, must be relieved without an undesirable increase in carbon dioxide.

The oxygen dissociation curve (Fig. 8-1) can help to explain the physiologic principle of controlled oxygen therapy. For a very small increase in arterial P_{O_2}, oxygen saturation can be increased significantly, with the result that more oxygen is available for delivery to the tissues. Therefore the inspired oxygen concentration need be raised only to a level that will bring arterial P_{O_2} and saturation within a safe physiologic range.

Normally, the inspired oxygen concentration of ambient air is 21%, which at sea level gives a partial pressure of 150 mm Hg. In controlled oxygen therapy an adequate oxygen saturation is usually achieved by increasing the patient's inspired oxygen concentration between 2% and 7%, or between 15 and 53 mm Hg (2% of 760 mm Hg = 15 mm Hg). When a patient commences treatment initially, the oxygen concentration of the lowest percentage is administered. Provided that no significant increase in arterial carbon dioxide tension (there is usually some increase) is noted and that the patient is not relapsing into a comatose state, then further increases in oxygen concentration can be continued.

The patient requiring controlled oxygen therapy should be under constant observation and is a candidate for intensive respiratory nursing care. A factor that often predisposes an exacerbation of symptoms in patients with chronic lung disease is infection, which results in an increase in pulmonary secretions and inhibition of adequate alveolar ventilation. Controlled oxygen therapy will do nothing to improve this condition. Only good nursing care with vigorous treatment for the removal of secretions can accomplish this. Nursing observations must include the signs and symptoms of carbon dioxide retention (Chapter 9).

Methods of oxygen administration

Numerous methods are now available for the administration of oxygen therapy. Some of the more common types of equipment in use are masks, cannulas, catheters, and tents. When oxygen is given, the method chosen should be selected with four things in mind: (1) the level of inspired oxygen achieved by the method, (2) the accuracy of control of the oxygen concentration, (3) patient comfort, and (4) patient expense.

Oxygen is supplied in many facilities from a central source and is piped to wall outlets at the patient's bedside. Tanks containing oxygen are used as a supply source when the pipeline system is not available. The disadvantages of tanks are that they are cumbersome and that the supply can run out, which may go unnoticed. Accurate valves and flowmeters are necessary to control the oxygen concentration delivered from any source, and a method for humidification of the oxygen inspired must be located between the flowmeter and the patient. Dry oxygen should never be given to a patient.

Oxygen masks may be divided into two main types: (1) masks that deliver high concentrations of oxygen and (2) masks that deliver low concentrations of oxygen. It might be reasoned that whatever flow setting is seen on the flowmeter should reflect the amount of oxygen that the patient is inspiring, but masks vary tremendously in the actual amount of oxygen they deliver to the patient.

The *simple face mask*, which is made of plastic, is lightweight, fairly comfortable, disposable, and has no reservoir bag. It is commonly used for oxygen administration in short-term therapy; for example, in the early postoperative period or when intermittent oxygen therapy is required. Patients tolerate the mask well, but it has disadvanages. It is loose fitting and therefore leaks, and it delivers oxygen concentrations anywhere from 35% to 60%. The concentration is difficult to regulate, and therefore the mask is undesirable for the patient with carbon dioxide retention. Oxygen concentration is achieved by rates of oxygen flow between 6 to 10 liters/min. Lower flow rates of oxygen cannot be used because for pure oxygen to be inspired, rates of oxygen flow should equal or be higher than the patient's minute ventilation.

Nasal cannulas are another simple, comfortable way of delivering oxygen to a patient (Fig. 8-2). Two cannulas, about ½ inch long, protrude from the center of a disposable semicircular tube and are inserted into the nostrils. An oxygen inlet is on the side of the tube, where variable concentrations of oxygen can be administered to the patient. At flow rates of 6 liters/min a concentration of 40% oxygen is achieved; from 60% to 70% concentrations are achieved with 10 liter/min flows. If nasal cannulas are used for patients with chronic alveolar hypoventilation and carbon dioxide retention, rates of flow should not exceed *1 to 2 liters/min* until arterial blood gas results are obtained. Chief advantages of this method are that the cannulas are inexpensive and the patient does not have to remove the device when he eats, talks, laughs, coughs, or does breathing exercises.

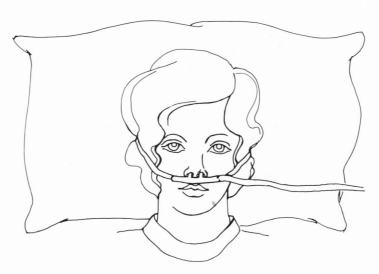

FIG. 8-2. Nasal cannulas.

A common place to find the face mask or the nasal cannulas is on a patient's fore-head, a chief disadvantage. Patients should be discouraged from displacing this equipment.

A *nonrebreathing mask* should be used if high concentrations of oxygen are to be delivered accurately. This is a tight-fitting mask, usually of rubber with a reservoir bag and a nonrebreathing valve. Oxygen flows into the bag and mask during inhalation, and a one-way valve between the bag and face mask prevents exhaled air from flowing back into the bag where it could be rebreathed. The exhaled air escapes instead through a one-way flap valve in the center of the mask. Although most efficient, this is an uncomfortable way of receiving oxygen. The mask of rubber is kept in position by a rubber harness, and the whole piece of equipment feels hot and sticky within a short time. Concentrations of 95% oxygen can be obtained by this method, which is most valuable in the acute stages of myocardial infarction.

A *plastic face mask with reservoir bag* (Fig. 8-3) is a commonly used method for delivering oxygen. This type of equipment is made of disposable, lightweight plastic, and many such masks have a partial rebreathing valve. Although a portion of the exhaled air passes into the reservoir bag, the amount of fresh oxygen in the bag far outweighs any effect of exhaled carbon dioxide. Rebreathing carbon dioxide could be a problem only if the reservoir bag is not kept inflated. A concentration of 70% oxygen can be obtained by this method, with oxygen flow rates of 10 liters/min.

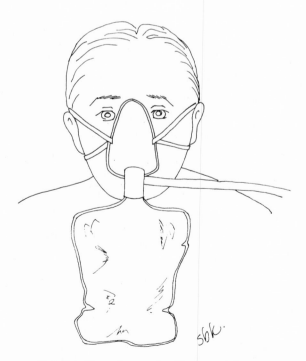

FIG. 8-3. Plastic face mask with reservoir bag.

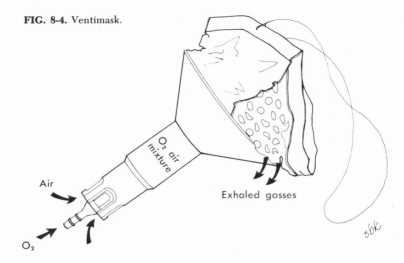

FIG. 8-4. Ventimask.

The *Ventimask* (Fig. 8-4) is a most important contribution to respiratory medicine. It is developed from the original venturi mask designed by Dr. E. J. M. Campbell for patients with chronic alveolar hypoventilation and carbon dioxide retention. The principles of physics developed by Venturi (1822) are utilized, and oxygen is delivered through a small jet in the center of a wide-bore cone at the base of the mask. As oxygen flows through the narrow jet, air is entrained, or pulled, through openings in the cone. This is demonstrated by the arrows in Fig. 8-4. The mask vents through which exhaled gas escapes are also shown.

Controlled oxygen therapy is attained with the Ventimask or a Mix-O-Mask, which incorporates the venturi principle of air entrainment. An air-oxygen mixture reaches the patient with the desired oxygen concentration. Four separate Ventimasks are available to deliver 24%, 28%, 35%, and 40% oxygen, with oxygen flow rates of 4, 6, 8, and 10 liters/min respectively.* Mix-O-Masks are available to deliver also 24%, 28%, 35%, and 40% oxygen, with oxygen flow rates of 4 liters/min for the two masks of lower concentration and 8 liters/min for the 35% and 40% masks.

These masks were designed so that the patient would receive the amount of oxygen stated within ±1% at the flow rates indicated. Researchers have found, however, the variance to be ±2%, with the 24% Ventimask delivering a 2% higher concentration.

There are two minor disadvantages of the Ventimask. One is that a thin elastic secures the mask in position, which cuts into the skin behind the ears. A wad of gauze under each side of the elastic will prevent this discomfort. A second disadvantage, as with all masks, is that the device must be removed when the patient eats.

The *oropharyngeal catheter* ("nasal catheter") provides another route for oxygen administration, and concentrations of up to 50% oxygen can be achieved by this

---

*Manufacturers recommend that the flow rates for the 28% Ventimask and the 40% Ventimask should be 4 and 8 liters/min, respectively; studies, however, have indicated that the flow rates of 6 and 10 liters/min are needed for the desired concentration to be delivered.

method. The effectiveness of the oropharyngeal catheter as a route for oxygen administration and the fact that it does not have to be removed for the patient to take nourishment have long been held as the virtues over other methods. Now, however, there seems to be little doubt that nasal cannulas are as effective, are more comfortable, and are far better tolerated by the patient with fewer complications.

Oxygen tents are used with decreasing frequency in adult hospital practice and prove to be of limited value when the canopy has to be entered frequently (for example, for monitoring vital signs every 15 minutes). The oxygen concentration is variable and difficult to control. Rates of flow of 20 liters/min are required to achieve a concentration of 60%, which immediately falls once the tent is opened.

Positive end expiratory pressure (PEEP) is being used with increasing frequency in improving oxygenation in the patient with severe hypoxemia that is unresponsive to treatment with high concentrations of oxygen: for example, a patient undergoing assisted ventilation who has an arterial PO_2 of 60 mm Hg while receiving 100% oxygen (normal 580 mm Hg).

It has been found that PEEP prevents the collapse of terminal airways and keeps the alveoli open at the end of expiration, thus enabling more oxygen uptake at the alveolar capillary surface.

The therapeutic importance of PEEP is that it allows for a reduction in the inspired oxygen concentration, thus preventing complications caused by long exposure to high concentrations of oxygen.

Success of oxygen therapy depends on continued, uninterrupted administration of oxygen during the treatment period. This is necessary to maintain adequate levels of arterial PO_2 and to prevent hypoxia. Erratic oxygen administration is unsatisfactory and is best avoided. When a patient's condition has improved and oxygen administration is to be discontinued, the patient should be weaned off oxygen by gradual reduction of the concentration inspired until the PO_2 is at an optimum level.

REFERENCES

Andrews, J. L., Jr.: Physiology and treatment of hypoxia, Clin. Notes Respir. Dis. **13:**3-14, 1974.

Bryan-Brown, C. W., Se-Min, B., Makabali, G., and Shoemaker, W. C.: Consumable oxygen: availability of oxygen in relation to oxyhemoglobin dissociation, Crit. Care Med. **1:**17-21, 1973.

Campbell, E. J. M., and Gebbie, T.: Masks and tents for providing controlled oxygen concentrations, Lancet **1:**468-469, 1966.

Finch, C. A., and Lenfant, C.: Oxygen transport in man, N. Engl. J. Med. **286:**407-416, 1972.

Friedman, S. A., Weber, B., Briscoe, W. A., Smith, J. P., and King, T. K.: Oxygen therapy: evaluation of various air-entraining masks, J.A.M.A. **228:**474-478, 1974.

Laurenzi, G. A., Sam, Y., and Guarneri, J. J.: Adverse effect on tracheal mucus flow, N. Engl. J. Med. **279:**333-343, 1968.

Linman, J.: Physiologic and pathophysiologic effects of anemia, N. Engl. J. Med. **279:**812-818, 1968.

Lorrain-Smith, J.: Pathological effects due to increase in oxygen tension in air breathed, J. Physiol. **24:**19-35, 1899.

Ngai, S. H., editor: Symposium on oxygen, Anesthesiology **37:**99-260, 1972.

Scottish Health Services Council: Uses and dangers of oxygen therapy, Edinburgh, 1969, Her Majesty's Stationery Office.

Singer, M. M., Wright, F., Stanley, L. K., Roe, B. B., and Hamilton, W. K.: Oxygen toxicity in man: a prospective study in patients after open heart surgery, N. Engl. J. Med. **283:**1473-1478, 1970.

Whipp, B. J.: Hypoxia and the control of ventilation, Respir. Ther., pp. 59-62, Nov./Dec., 1972.

9 / RESPIRATORY FAILURE

Patients with acute respiratory failure require all the professional and technical skills the nurse possesses, since these patients do not have just one disease entity but many. This is clearly demonstrated by the variety of patients admitted to an intensive respiratory care unit. Whether the patient has burns or a chronic obstructive pulmonary disease, he may experience respiratory failure, and the nurse must know how the respiratory apparatus works to understand how it can fail. This chapter shows how the respiratory physiology previously presented can be readily applied to this end.

GENERAL CONSIDERATIONS
Respiratory failure defined

The current, most widely accepted definition of respiratory failure is *the inability of the respiratory apparatus to maintain adequate oxygenation of the blood, with or without carbon dioxide retention.* Impairment of gas exchange is the major factor in respiratory failure and is of two distinct types: (1) *hypoxemic respiratory failure,* with a reduction in arterial Po_2 (60 mm Hg or below) and a normal or slightly decreased arterial Pco_2; or (2) *hypoventilatory respiratory failure* characterized, as the name implies, by both hypoxemia and an elevated arterial Pco_2 (>50 mm Hg) (hypercapnia).

Causes of respiratory failure

Normal blood gases are maintained by the balance and integrity of ventilation, blood flow, and diffusion. Should any of these processes fail, the result will be impairment in gas exchange, which may progress to respiratory failure. In patients with *normal lungs* hypoventilatory respiratory failure is most likely (not always) to develop with decreased respiratory drive or neuromuscular disorders. The adult respiratory distress syndrome results in severe hypoxemic respiratory failure and is discussed in Chapter 10.

If the lungs are *abnormal,* airways obstruction, thoracic deformity, or impaired diaphragmatic movement may result in hypoventilatory failure, and impaired diffusion is most likely to predispose hypoxemic respiratory failure. Because there is often a complex derangement of body systems, the causes of respiratory failure are not always clear cut. What may start off as being essentially a hypoxemic condition may become hypoventilatory or vice versa, with a good sprinkling of possible metabolic disturbances to confuse the situation. (See Table 10.)

TABLE 10. Some causes of respiratory failure

Normal lungs	Abnormal lungs and/or thorax

1. Decreased respiratory drive
   a. Drug intoxication
   b. Anesthetic agents
   c. Cerebral trauma – tumour – ↑ ICP
   d. Severe metabolic
     alkalosis
   e. Cardiac arrest
2. Neuromuscular disorders
   a. Spinal injury
   b. Guillain-Barré syndrome
   c. Myasthenia gravis
   d. Multiple sclerosis
3. Adult respiratory
  distress syndrome
   a. Shock
   b. Prolonged respirator therapy
   c. Prolonged O_2 therapy
   d. Fat embolism
   e. Pulmonary contusion
   f. Fluid overload
   g. Pulmonary emboli
   h. Diffuse "capillary
     leak" syndrome
	1. Airways obstruction
	   a. Chronic bronchitis
	   b. Emphysema
	   c. Asthma
	   d. Tumor
	2. Thoracic deformity
	   a. Trauma (flail chest)
	   b. Surgical incision
	   c. Kyphoscoliosis
	   d. Pectus excavatum
	3. Impaired diaphragmatic
	  movement
	   a. Trauma
	   b. Paralysis
	4. Impaired diffusion
	   a. Pulmonary fibrosis
	   b. Radiation pneumonitis
	   c. Pulmonary emboli
	   d. Destruction of pulmonary
	     capillary bed

Diagnosis of respiratory failure

A diagnosis of respiratory failure is made using three parameters: (1) a history of a condition that may predispose respiratory failure, (2) clinical manifestations, (3) measurement of arterial blood gases and pH. Since the major factor in respiratory failure is impairment of gas exchange, arterial blood gas analysis will always be the deciding factor when confirming the diagnosis. The type of failure (hypoxemic or hypoventilatory) can be determined by blood gas measurements; many evaluations of pulmonary function, such as physiologic dead space (VD), alveolar-arterial oxygen tension differences (A-aDO_2), and true shunts also require measurements of arterial blood gases (Chapter 11).

Clinical manifestations of respiratory failure

When respiratory failure occurs acutely as a result of obstruction of a major airway or cardiac arrest, changes in the patient's condition are dramatic and overt. In many instances, however, the clinical features are more subtle and include hypoxemia, hypercapnia, hypotension, or dyspnea. As the nurse will recall, the signs and symptoms of hypoxemia and hypoxia are not easily recognized, and these plus the other clinical manifestations may be masked by a number of conditions that may or may not predispose respiratory failure. These are important clinical entities, however, and the nurse should make the effort to identify them.

Hypercapnia. Normally adequate alveolar ventilation maintains an arterial P_{CO_2} of 40 mm Hg by eliminating approximately 200 ml of carbon dioxide each minute. This is usually equal to the amount of carbon dioxide produced in the tissues. An important factor is that the level of carbon dioxide in arterial blood is inversely proportional to alveolar ventilation; in other words, if alveolar ventilation is halved, arterial P_{CO_2} will be doubled. Thus when alveolar ventilation is inadequate to remove the carbon dioxide produced, the partial pressure of carbon dioxide will rise.

The major effect of marked increases in carbon dioxide tensions in body fluids is depression of the central nervous system, reflected by drowsiness and inability to concentrate and a gradual, progressive loss of consciousness. In patients with respiratory failure these changes occur rapidly and may go completely unnoticed, but there are certain classic warning signs that the nurse at the bedside may observe as significant manifestations of hypercapnia.

Studies of the effects of gradual increases in arterial carbon dioxide levels have been performed on subjects with normal lungs and cerebral function. These studies were conducted under controlled conditions where the nursing staff or the subjects involved were not aware of the gradual increases in P_{CO_2}. The subjects studied were given carbon dioxide in 40% oxygen in sufficient amounts over a period of 5 days to gradually increase their arterial P_{CO_2} from normal up to 75 mm Hg. The first signs observed were drowsiness, the inability of the subjects to concentrate, and confusion. These signs were accompanied by irritability with the nursing staff, general dissatisfaction with nursing care, hospital food, and so on. The subjects complained of headache and an inability to sleep. This is thought to be related to cerebral vasodilatation that occurs with increases in carbon dioxide levels and a resulting increase in the pressure of cerebrospinal fluid.

It is not uncommon for patients with carbon dioxide retention to have a reversal in their sleep patterns; they may be drowsy through the day and wide awake at night. This, accompanied by the signs and symptoms mentioned, often results in such patients being labeled difficult and cranky. If these manifestations are unrecognized as symptoms of hypercapnia, sedation may be administered to a patient, which would depress the respiratory center and result in further increases in arterial P_{CO_2}—followed by coma and death. Carbon dioxide narcosis is usually *induced* either by uncontrolled oxygen therapy or sedation, particularly tranquilizers. The nurse should always keep these facts in mind when caring for respiratory patients with hypercapnia.

Hypoxia and hypoxemia. In patients with respiratory failure major factors are hypoxia and hypoxemia. Normal relationships of ventilation, blood flow, and diffusion maintain an arterial P_{O_2} of 90 to 100 mm Hg at sea level with an inspired oxygen concentration of 150 mm Hg. The alveolar P_{O_2} is determined by the arterial P_{CO_2} and the inspired oxygen concentration. Hypoxemia may be acute or chronic.

Acute hypoxemia may result from sudden airway obstruction, circulatory failure, blockage of alveoli by fluid as in pulmonary edema, or severe hemorrhage. Clinical manifestations may include headache, euphoria, and impaired motor function—symptoms that may progress to delirium and unconsciousness. "Air hunger" is seen in some instances where the patient gulps to get sufficient air. The initial cardiovascular responses to acute hypoxemia are hypertension, tachycardia, and an increased cardiac output. As the condition continues, the blood pressure falls and central cyanosis manifests itself.

Chronic hypoxemia is a progressive condition that is present in patients with chronic lung disease and certain types of cardiovascular disease. In the presence of persistent hypoxemia, the body makes an attempt to compensate so that adequate oxygen can be delivered to the tissues. Chronic hypoxemia causes stimulation of the bone marrow to produce more red cells, which results in a secondary polycythemia and thus more hemoglobin to carry oxygen. This same phenomenon is found in subjects who adapt to a high altitude environment, where the reduction in oxygen concentration in the inspired air causes hypoxemia (Chapter 8).

Cyanosis may be present in acute or chronic hypoxia. The degree of cyanosis is determined by the amount of reduced hemoglobin circulating in the blood. The unsaturated hemoglobin gives the bluish discoloration to the skin and mucous membranes. Since the arterial oxygen saturation must be as low as 78% before cyanosis becomes apparent, this condition is not a useful sign for the early detection of hypoxemia. If present, cyanosis requires immediate treatment with oxygen therapy.

The tissues most affected by hypoxia are those of the central nervous system and the myocardium. Body stores of oxygen are extremely limited, and complete cessation of breathing from respiratory arrest will result in death from hypoxia within approximately 4 minutes. This limited amount of time is all it takes for body stores of oxygen to be depleted when a patient is breathing air. Some patients in respiratory failure will already have a reduced oxygen supply to the brain and myocardium because of impairment in local circulation (cerebral and coronary); this will further increase the dangers of hypoxemia.

MANAGEMENT OF PATIENTS IN RESPIRATORY FAILURE

Management of patients in respiratory failure depends on the cause and type of failure. The main objective in hypoventilatory respiratory failure is to restore adequate alveolar ventilation. In hypoxemic failure the objective is to give sufficient oxygen to relieve the hypoxemia and prevent hypoxia without causing further damage to an already injured lung. Certain general principles of treatment, however, are applied in both instances and include the following:

1. Airway patency
2. Oxygen therapy
3. Adequate ventilation
4. Drug therapy
5. Hydration
6. Removal of secretions
7. Prevention of infection
8. Rehabilitation

Airway patency

Establishment and maintenance of an open airway is of critical importance in management of patients in respiratory failure. Blockage by a foreign body or plug of mucus can result in sudden respiratory collapse and death if the object causing the obstruction is not removed. When spontaneous respirations are present, an *oropharyngeal airway* can be used. This prevents the tongue from falling back and thus blocking the upper airway, and it provides a route for aspiration of oropharyngeal secretions. This method is most commonly used to maintain airway patency during the postanesthesia period or when a patient lapses intermittently into semiconsciousness, as he may do following drug overdosage or neurologic disturbances.

Endotracheal intubation. The method most widely used to institute and maintain an open airway is endotracheal intubation by either the nasal or oral route. A physician deciding which route to use will consider (1) local preference, (2) the duration of intubation, (3) the degree of emergency, (4) available equipment, and (5) the age of the patient. For long-term intubation (a week or more) and in children the nasal route is often selected. It permits better fixation of the tube and is more easily tolerated in the conscious patient. Intubation by way of the oral route may be selected for emergency short-term use, as in anesthesia or resuscitation.

Chief advantages. Endotracheal intubation has several advantages. It provides a route for short-term mechanical ventilation and thus often obviates the need for tracheostomy. Endotracheal intubation protects the lower respiratory tract from aspirated material (vomitus or secretions), and it facilitates the removal of pulmonary secretions. The advantages are of particular value in the following situations: (1) in cardiopulmonary resuscitation, (2) during the early postoperative period when patients have undergone major cardiovascular surgery, (3) to relieve carbon dioxide retention in acute exacerbations of pulmonary disease, and (4) in the prevention and treatment of acute respiratory failure.

The length of time that an endotracheal tube is left in situ is a topic for constant debate and rests entirely with the physicians managing the patient. With recent improvements in materials used to manufacture endotracheal tubes, there appears to be less chance of irritation of the respiratory mucosa. This has led to the practice in some facilities of leaving an endotracheal tube in position for up to 2 weeks. A more conservative period of 7 days or less is, however, more generally accepted.

Endotracheal tubes. There are many types of endotracheal tubes. They are usually constructed of rubber or plastic and are available in a number of sizes with or without an inflatable cuff. The size of the tube is an important consideration when a patient is to be intubated, whether the nasal or the oral route is used. Because airways resistance is increased in long narrow tubes, the physician will generally choose the largest tube that a patient can safely tolerate.

Care of the patient undergoing endotracheal intubation. When the patient to be intubated is conscious, the necessity for the treatment is explained to the patient and his immediate family by the patient's physician. The nurse should explain the procedure, making sure that the patient understands that he will be unable to speak. The nurse should reassure him that someone will always be with him and that he will be kept as comfortable as possible. The patient must also be shown new methods by which he can communicate. Topical and local anesthetic agents should be applied to the route of intubation (for example, 4 to 5 ml of 4% lignocaine spray to the gums, tongue, and pharynx or cocaine hydrochloride to the nose).

The equipment required for endotracheal intubation includes endotracheal tubes of various sizes, a laryngoscope with a selection of different-sized blades, lubricant, topical and local anesthetic agents, Magill forceps, gauze swabs, adhesive tape, and plastic syringes. In addition, equipment for oxygenation, ventilation, and cardiac resuscitation should be available.

It is the nurse's responsibility to check the cuffs on the endotracheal tubes *prior to* use and to lubricate the selected tube. The laryngoscope light must be working; batteries and extra bulbs should be at hand; and suction equipment must also be working.

Nursing patients with an endotracheal tube in situ includes many techniques employed when nursing the tracheostomized patient (p. 147). Special consideration is given to the length and type of suction catheter used. The catheter must be of an adequate length to traverse the length of the endotracheal tube and enter the left and right main bronchus in order for secretions to be removed effectively.

Complications. Complications that may arise at the time of endotracheal intubation include faulty placement of the tube (for example, in the right main stem bronchus), obstruction of the tube by a plug of mucus, or trauma to the larynx during the procedure resulting in severe spasm and laryngeal edema. Minor irritation to the larynx will produce spasm and edema, and if it is to be avoided, endotracheal intubation should be conducted by a skilled person; an anesthesiologist should be called when the need for a patient to be intubated arises.

Prolonged endotracheal intubation most commonly results in laryngeal damage. In less serious cases this is demonstrated by hoarseness for 2 to 24 hours after extubation. In certain instances laryngeal edema occurs, which may result in severe stridor that develops 2 to 3 hours following extubation and is often serious enough for the patient to be reintubated and treated with steroid therapy. Tube pressure may result in a complication known as subglottic stenosis. The seriousness of complications arising from endotracheal intubation appear to be directly related to the length of time that a patient has the tube in situ.

Tracheostomy. Another method of securing and maintaining an open airway is by surgical incision and intubation of the trachea (tracheostomy). This may be a temporary or permanent opening into the trachea; the latter usually follows laryngectomy. There are five main indications for tracheostomy, some of which overlap those for endotracheal intubation:

1. Obstruction in the upper respiratory tract (for example, by laryngeal edema, burns, or neoplasm)
2. To provide an open airway in patients with conditions that are expected to persist longer than the period considered safe for endotracheal intubation (for example, Guillain-Barré syndrome)
3. Removal of secretions from the trachea and bronchi when this has not been possible with physiotherapy and intubation
4. Prevention of aspiration of secretions or vomitus from the pharynx into the lower respiratory tract
5. To provide a route for mechanical ventilation

Whenever endotracheal intubation is not feasible (for example, in the circumstances listed under 1 and 2), a tracheostomy should be performed and is generally conducted as an elective procedure in the operating room with an endotracheal tube in situ. An emergency tracheostomy is usually performed only when an insurmountable obstruction is present in the upper airway. The advantages of tracheostomy as elective surgery are that the patient and his relatives can be prepared for the procedure and that prior endotracheal intubation provides a route for adequate ventilation, oxygen delivery, and aspiration of secretions prior to and during the procedure.

Technique. A transverse, U-shaped surgical incision is usually made into the trachea at the level of the second or third tracheal ring. This is known as a high tracheostomy and is performed in order to keep the tracheostomy tube above the carina, thus lessening the risk of the tube entering the right main stem bronchus. Following skin suture and tracheal aspiration, a tracheostomy tube of the correct size, with the cuff checked, is slipped into position and secured with tapes around the patient's neck.

Tracheostomy tubes. There are many types of tracheostomy tubes available. Tubes are made of plastic or other synthetic material, rubber, and silver. Plastic tracheostomy tubes are being used most frequently today in treating respiratory failure. Their advantages are (1) they are built with a much sharper angle, which provides a better fit; (2) they are malleable yet do not kink or disintegrate with use; and (3) they have a built-in cuff. Many plastic tubes are used without an inner cannula and have proved to be most satisfactory when adequate humidification is provided.

Precautionary measures involved when selecting a tracheostomy tube include the size of the tube, the choice between metal and plastic, the inflation of the cuff, and the use of inner cannulas.

Like the endotracheal tube the tracheostomy tube should be as large as the trachea will tolerate. As the airway is narrowed, airway resistance increases (Chapter 4), and additional pressure is required to overcome this resistance for ventilation to be adequate.

If a patient is receiving radiation therapy to the neck, a metal tracheostomy tube should not be inserted because of the additional "scattering" of rays outside the prescribed area. In these circumstances the plastic tube may be used, but it should be replaced following each treatment because radiation causes chemical changes to the tube, which make it tissue toxic.

Overinflation of the built-in cuff on plastic tracheostomy tubes can cause herniation of the cuff over the end of the tube, which will cause acute obstruction of the trachea. This is a particular danger where the cuff has a high residual volume and has to be deflated prior to each inflation.

Tracheostomy cuffs. To prevent damage to the tracheal wall (one of the major complications following tracheostomy), much attention has been given to the design, manufacture, and use of tracheostomy cuffs. Ideally tracheostomy cuffs should (1) expand evenly, (2) have a high residual volume, (3) be oblong in shape, (4) be floppy in texture, and (5) have a low intracuff pressure. These combinations are important so that the inflated cuff conforms to the tracheal wall rather than distorting it. Low-pressure cuffs provide this; these advantages are lost, however, if the cuff is overinflated.

To prevent overinflation of tracheostomy cuffs, many tubes are now available with a pressure-controlled inflation valve, which is usually located in the pilot balloon. This prevents the cuff pressure from exceeding 25 cm H_2O—the pressure suggested for the minimal occluding volume (MOV) discussed later.

Care of the patient with a tracheostomy. Constant skilled medical and nursing management, involving the application of many aspects of respiratory physiology, is important to the care of the tracheostomized patient. Initially the patient is frightened, frustrated, and completely dependent on members of the health team, particularly the nursing staff. The nurse caring for the patient with a tracheostomy should be fully aware of why the procedure was necessary, and should be in a position to reassure and give support to the patient and his family. Expert nursing care may be given keeping the following guidelines in mind:

1. Humidification
2. Communication
3. Explanation
4. Observation
5. Asepsis
6. Aspiration
7. Cuff inflation and deflation
8. Rehabilitation

Important structures are bypassed when a tracheostomy is performed. These include the normal air-conditioning unit provided by the upper respiratory tract and the larynx and the glottis. When the normal function of the upper respiratory tract is interrupted by tracheostomy or endotracheal intubation, adequate humidification is essential at all times, whether or not the patient is receiving ventilatory assistance. Addition of moisture to the inspired air is vital in preventing drying and crusting of secretions and aiding in liquefaction of tenacious sputum.

Warmed and moistened gas mist (either compressed air or oxygen) may be continuously supplied to a patient with a tracheostomy by way of a lightweight tracheostomy mask (Fig. 9-1). This is a well-fitting mask and has a swivel inlet for the humidified gas, which allows the patient freedom of movement. Suctioning can be carried out through the center port without removing the mask from the patient. The T-piece shown in Fig. 9-2 serves the same function as the tracheostomy mask but is also used

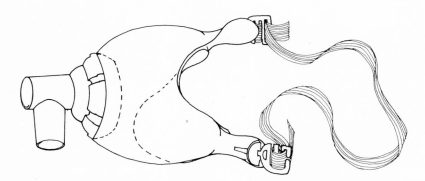

FIG. 9-1. Tracheostomy mask, used for humidification of inspired gas. Inlet (left) swivels to give the patient freedom of movement.

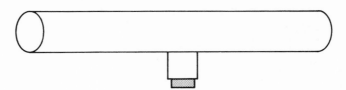

FIG. 9-2. The T-piece is designed to provide a free flow of humidified gas through the cylindrical portion, which the patient receives by way of the center connection.

in patients with an endotracheal tube in situ. Its lightweight construction of plastic prevents the T-piece from dragging on the endotracheal tube and causing the patient discomfort. When a constant mist or fog is seen coming from the T-piece or tracheostomy mask, humidification is adequate. Water frequently collects in the tubes that connect the delivery systems to their source of humidification, and these should be checked and emptied frequently.

Most frightening to the patient with a tracheostomy is the inability to speak. He cannot ask a question or call for help. Reassurance and constant attendance alleviate much of this fear, but methods for the patient to communicate must be provided. A hand bell or other device loud enough to attract attention should be within the patient's reach. A spoon tied to each bed rail works very well. Also on hand should be scratch pads and pencils and a series of flash cards with requests commonly made by patients printed on them.

Functions that require a forced expiration against a closed glottis, such as coughing and defecation, cannot be carried out as effectively by the patient with a tracheostomy, since the glottis is bypassed. Laryngeal and glottic function are restored when the cuff on a tracheostomy tube is deflated and the tube is plugged. This allows for the normal passage of air through the upper respiratory tract and over the vocal chords.

Tracheostomy care requires the use of strict aseptic nursing techniques when handling the tracheostomy wound, the tracheostomy tube, or any piece of equipment that is attached to or comes into contact with the tracheal stoma. Care includes the following:

1. Dressing of the tracheostomy wound should be frequent and may be necessary several times during a shift. A soiled tracheostomy dressing will predispose wound infection, which may then result in infection of the trachea and respiratory tract. It is rather like having a dirty doormat and a clean hallway.

2. Removal, cleansing, and sterilization of the inner cannula (if used) every 4 hours is necessary to prevent secretions from collecting around and blocking the end of the tracheostomy tube.

3. Sterile gloves and equipment must be used when aspirating tracheobronchial secretions.

4. Secretions should *always* be suctioned from the pharynx *prior to* cuff deflation. *Never* use the same catheter for this purpose as for removing tracheobronchial secretions.

5. Any piece of equipment, such as a ventilator attachment, which is disconnected temporarily from the tracheostomy during tracheal aspiration should be placed on a sterile paper towel (not on the patient's chest or bedclothes) during the procedure.

Suctioning techniques. The removal of secretions with a tracheostomy or endo-tracheal tube must be aseptic, atraumatic, and effective. *Asepsis* is accomplished by using a freshly opened sterile suction catheter, which is handled with sterile gloves or a sterile instrument as it is guided into the right then left main bronchus. The catheters should not be left standing in solution or cleared with a solution and then reused. Any equipment that connects directly to the endotracheal or trache-ostomy tube must be placed on a sterile field during suctioning.

Removal of secretions should be as atraumatic as possible to the patient. Damage to the delicate respiratory structures and oxygen depletion during the procedure must be avoided. The catheter used should be sufficiently long to enter the right and left main bronchi. It should have an open end and side holes (whistle tip) and be of a smooth, pliable material yet be firm enough not to collapse when suction is applied. A curved-tipped catheter facilitates suctioning of the left main bronchus.

The side vent on most catheters allows thumb control of suction during the re-moval of secretions. To avoid trauma, suction should *never* be applied during inser-tion of the catheter but only during its withdrawal. Secretions are removed by rotating the catheter between the thumb and forefinger as it is removed, not by moving the catheter up and down.

To prevent hypoxia in the already hypoxemic patient, particularly patients with large amounts of "shunting," preoxygenation and postoxygenation for a few breaths with 100% oxygen may be required. To avoid hypoxia, suctioning of any patient should be limited to 15 seconds with adequate reoxygenation of the patient between times.

To avoid excessive intrathoracic negative pressure, the pressure of the suction apparatus should not be above 80 to 100 mm Hg.

Effective suctioning is accomplished by removing secretions from the right and left main bronchi. Unless the catheter is long enough, this is difficult to accomplish with a nasoendotracheal tube. To guide the catheter into either bronchus, the patient's head is turned away from the direction in which the nurse is proceeding (head turned to the left for entering the right main bronchus, head turned to the right for entering the left main bronchus). Because the angle of the left main bronchus is sharp, catheter entry is often difficult. Some people believe that turning of the patient's head is of little or no advantage; I find, however, that it works for me.

Instillation of normal saline into the respiratory tract may be necessary to liquefy and mobilize secretions. Usually the violent coughing reaction that the patient has will dislodge a considerable amount of mucus. Between 5 to 10 ml of sterile normal saline is instilled into the trachea from a sterile syringe (without the needle) prior to suc-tioning. Most patients dislike the sensation of suffocation or drowning they feel from direct instillation of fluids into the trachea, but it is a most effective way of loosening stubborn mucus.

Cuff inflation and deflation. There have been many changes in opinion with regard to the need for regular cuff deflation (5 minutes each hour) as a means of preventing tracheal wall damage. The theory is that cuff deflation allows return of the circulation to the tracheal mucosa, thus preventing tissue necrosis from tissue ischemia. The consensus at the time of writing is that patients who can tolerate being off a ventilator for 5 to 10 minutes should have the cuff deflated on an hourly basis or that the cuff should be deflated when a patient requires suctioning. The nurse must remember always to remove the secretions from the pharynx prior to cuff deflation.

When the cuff is inflated, it should only be inflated to the minimal occluding volume (MOV). That is the minimal amount of air required to inflate the cuff to provide an airtight seal during mechanical ventilation (some patients can tolerate a slight leak). As the cuff is slowly inflated during positive pressure inspiration, listen for air leak. Stop inflating the cuff at the minimum amount at which (1) no air leak is detected, (2) the patient is unable to phonate, (3) the ventilator stops hissing and will trigger inspiration, and (4) no air leak is felt around the nose, mouth, or tracheostomy stoma. This volume should not exceed 25 cm H_2O (18 mm Hg), which is measured at the pilot balloon with a pressure manometer. The pressure is measured at the end of exhalation and should always be recorded each time the cuff has to be reinflated. An increase in the MOV may indicate a faulty cuff or one with a slow leak. It may also indicate structural changes in the tracheal wall due to damage.

Complications. At the time of the surgical procedure, the complications that may arise from tracheostomy include hemorrhage, misplacement of the tube in prebronchial tissue (resulting in surgical emphysema), or cardiopulmonary collapse. If a patient is suddenly overventilated, the rapid reduction in P_{CO_2} that follows not uncommonly predisposes ventricular fibrillation, thought to result from sudden changes in intracellular potassium levels. Should the arterial P_{CO_2} be lowered prior to adequate oxygenation, the patient will become apneic, because of (1) the sudden removal of accumulated carbon dioxide in the body, (2) cerebral vasoconstriction, and (3) hypoxia. These complications are reduced greatly when adequate ventilation is established by way of an endotracheal tube prior to the operative procedure.

In the first 4 to 5 days following the operation, decannulation may be a particular hazard because of the difficulties that may be encountered during reintubation. It takes about 5 days for the tracheostomy tube to form a well-defined pathway within the trachea, after which reintubation becomes easier. Decannulation is most likely to occur with coughing during cuff deflation. It is advisable therefore to have a second person hold the tracheostomy tube at the flange as the cuff is deflated and during suctioning at this time. There are many physicians who believe that cuff deflation should be avoided during the first 24 to 48 hours of the postoperative period to avoid the hazard of decannulation.

Equipment for reintubation should always be at the bedside of a patient with a tracheostomy, and nurses caring for these patients should be capable of replacing a tracheostomy tube in an emergency situation. The best way to learn this procedure is in a nonemergency situation under the guidance of a physician (for example, during routine tracheostomy tube changes). Equipment for tube replacement includes a sterile tracheostomy tube of the correct size with tapes in place, the cuff checked and the obturator in position, a tracheal dilator, scissors, hemostats, dressings, sterile towels, sterile gloves, and a syringe to inflate the cuff.

When a tracheostomy tube is to be replaced in a nonemergency situation, the procedure is explained to the patient and reassurance given. The patient is placed flat on his back in a head-down position to prevent aspiration of secretions from the pharynx. The pharynx is well suctioned and, if permitted, the patient is preoxygenated with 100% oxygen for a few minutes. All equipment is made ready. Immediately following removal of the old tube, the new tube is inserted through the stoma and directed well back toward the tracheal wall and passed downward in one smooth movement, then secured in position. A tracheal dilator may be required to open the wound a little wider to facilitate easier passage of the tube. A pediatric laryngoscope is often helpful in relocating the tract.

An obstructed tracheostomy tube is life threatening, and prompt action must be taken to establish a patient airway. When there is no physician at hand, the nurse should summon help, deflate the cuff, cut the tapes on the tube, remove the tube, insert a tracheal dilator to establish an airway, remove secretions, insert a new tube, and restore ventilaton.

Oxygen therapy

An adequate inspired Po_2 for one patient may not be adequate for another, and the underlying cause of the disorder must be examined. For most patients in respiratory failure, an inspired oxygen concentration that will maintain an arterial Po_2 close to the normal range (70 to 80 mm Hg) is the goal in management. Controlled low-flow oxygen therapy may always be administered safely and should be given to patients until the arterial blood gases have been analyzed and the cause of respiratory failure ascertained.

As shown in Chapter 8, oxygen uptake and transport are dependent on many factors. As a result, oxygen therapy does not guarantee the relief of hypoxia. When determining the effectiveness of oxygen therapy in patients, the physician will therefore evaluate certain components of the oxygen transport system. A patient's hemoglobin level will be measured to ascertain the quality of the oxygen-carrying capacity of the blood. Anemia, which is often present in hospitalized patients, results in a decrease in oxygen uptake and transport; it should be corrected if oxygen therapy is to be effective. Other factors to be considered are the adequacy of the "pump" and the "gas exchanger." In other words, is the heart working efficiently enough to maintain a normal cardiac output and distribution of blood flow through the pulmonary circulation and systemic circulation, and is alveolar ventilation being maintained at a level for gas exchange to be effective? Every effort is made to correct any defects in the oxygen transport system, and oxygen therapy is adjusted accordingly.

Adequate ventilation

The abnormalities in gas exchange incurred by inadequate alveolar ventilation are important features in the pattern of respiratory failure. Impairment may be severe enough to be life threatening, in which case ventilation must be assisted by mechanical means. There are many instances, however, when adequate ventilation can be restored following vigorous chest physiotherapy for the removal of secretions, the use of bronchodilators to relieve bronchospasm, and IPPB therapy to aerate underventilated alveoli.

Physiologic considerations. A review of normal ventilation, blood flow, and diffusion (Chapter 4) illustrates the interrelationships between cardiac and pulmonary mechanisms and the many factors that can alter the balance. To complicate matters in the patient undergoing mechanical ventilation, there is now the addition of a disease process and a machine to affect both pulmonary and cardiac function. Therefore a brief overview of the effects of mechanical ventilation on ventilation and circulation will be presented.

When mechanical ventilation is instituted, goals include improvement of total ventilation, improvement in alveolar ventilation, a better distribution of inspired gas, improvement in arterial blood gas tensions, and reduction of the patient's work in breathing. Achievement of a more normal and uniform distribution of inspired gas throughout the lung is a major advantage of positive-pressure breathing. This is accomplished with the opening of alveoli previously not involved in gas exchange. The result is improvement in overall alveolar ventilation, with concomitant improvement in ventilation-perfusion relationships. Once alveolar ventilation is improved, this will be reflected in the improvement of arterial blood gas tensions.

Normally we are not aware of the work of breathing, but patients with respiratory abnormalities frequently have to work hard to move a volume of air in or out of the lungs. This may be due to increased work required to move the thorax, the lungs, or the actual air itself (Chapter 4). When the work of breathing is effectively reduced by positive-pressure ventilation, the patient conserves energy and thus reduces oxygen consumption. Most importantly, he can rest.

Of major significance is the effect of mechanical ventilation on the cardiovascular system. During normal respiration, intrathoracic pressure is negative (subatmospheric) and becomes more so for air to flow into the lungs. As intrathoracic pressure falls during inspiration, venous return is enhanced to the right atrium which, in turn, increases right ventricular output and blood flow through the pulmonary capillaries. Passive exhalation reduces venous return as intrathoracic pressure returns to the resting level (−2 cm of water) and increases left atrial filling and left ventricular output. During positive-pressure ventilation normal processes are reversed. Positive pressure is applied during inspiration, which elevates the intrathoracic pressure above atmospheric. The expiratory phase then returns the intrathoracic pressure to atmospheric, not to the normal subatmospheric pressure. This occurs because the respiratory cycle during positive-pressure ventilation begins with a closed respiratory circuit between the patient's airways and the ventilator, the latter always returning to the pressure of the atmosphere.

The effect of mechanical ventilation on the cardiovascular system is also a reversal of normal function. Positive-pressure inhalation increases left atrial filling (temporarily) and exhalation increases venous return and right atrial filling. Subjecting the heart and blood vessels to increased intrathoracic pressures of even the smallest amount for more than the shortest time impairs venous return and cardiac output. To reduce these effects of mechanical ventilation, which may prove disastrous to the patient with cardiac abnormalities, the inspiratory phase of respiration should be kept as short as possible and the expiratory phase prolonged. This is termed the *inspiratory-expiratory time ratio* (I/E ratio) and is maintained where possible at 1:1.5 or 1:2.

Mechanical ventilation is defined as a mechanical device to augment respiratory gas flow. Machines most commonly used for this purpose fall into two main classifications—*pressure*-preset ventilators and *volume*-preset ventilators.

Since respiratory failure can occur in a variety of conditions, the ideal ventilator is one that will meet all the ventilatory needs of a patient and yet be durable, dependable, and easy to maintain. Modern ventilators, such as the Bennett MA-1 and the Ohio 560, may be used as volume preset or pressure preset and may be used in assisted or controlled ventilation. Breathing frequency and inspiratory and expiratory phases of ventilation can be varied to meet the individual needs of the patient. Adequate humidification and oxygen delivery over a wide variety of settings from room air to 100% may be achieved. A sigh mechanism is available to automatically hyperinflate a patient's lungs periodically.

Assisted ventilation. Assisted ventilation is used in patients who have spontaneous respiration but inadequate alveolar ventilation. When a ventilator is used to assist ventilation, it is set so that the patient triggers the machine on inspiration. A gas mixture is then delivered to the patient under increasing pressure, inflating the lungs until a preset pressure is reached. A valve is then opened, releasing the applied positive pressure, and exhalation occurs passively. This method of assisted ventilation is termed *patient cycled, pressure preset* and is satisfactory if high inflation pressures are *not* required to get an adequate volume of air into the lungs and if a patient's respiratory center is normally responsive. Normal lungs usually inflate at a pressure of 10 cm of water, and preset inflation pressures are usually set during assisted ventilation at 15 to 20 cm of water. In patients with obstructive pulmonary disease, inflation pressures of over 35 cm of water are often required to overcome reduced lung compliance and increased airways resistance.

Controlled ventilation. Controlled ventilation is used for patients with few or no spontaneous respirations. The machine is set at a predetermined respiratory cycle (rate, pressure, and tidal volume), which is delivered automatically by the machine. Patients requiring controlled ventilation (for example, those with Guillain-Barré syndrome or a spinal injury) often need it for a prolonged period.

Pressure-preset ventilators. Pressure-preset ventilators are designed to inflate a patient's lungs until a preset fixed pressure is reached, at which time inspiration ends and expiration begins. Pressure-preset ventilators may be time cycled (the breathing frequency is fixed) or patient cycled (the machine is triggered by the patient's breathing frequency).

Volume-preset ventilators. A fixed, uniform volume is delivered to patients with a volume-preset ventilator, which is usually set at a fixed rate. The advantage of a volume ventilator is that the preset volume will be delivered to the patient regardless of changes in airways resistance or compliance, providing that there is no leak in the system between the patient and the ventilator. Inflation pressures of between 80 and 100 cm of water can be delivered with a volume-preset ventilator.

Positive end expiratory pressure (PEEP). Positive end expiratory pressure may be used with or without mechanical ventilation. When PEEP is used with mechanical ventilation, the term frequently used is *continuous positive pressure ventilation* (CPPV).

By applying a pressure of between 5 and 15 cm H_2O during the end expiratory phase of respiration, alveoli and small airways that would normally collapse are held open. This provides for better distribution of ventilation with respect to blood flow throughout the lung, by increasing the functional residual capacity (FRC) (Chapter 3) with a subsequent reduction in venous admixture and hypoxemia.

Some mechanical ventilators come with a special expiratory valve for application of PEEP. If these are not available, one end of a piece of tubing is fitted to the exhalation port of the ventilator and the other end is then immersed under water to the desired level (5 to 15 cm H_2O).

Continuous positive airway pressure (CPAP). The term *CPAP* is used to mean PEEP applied without mechanical ventilation. Continuous positive airway pressure is maintained during spontaneous ventilation and is applied by way of a tube or face mask. The popularity of the use of CPAP with a head chamber in the newborn infant has led researchers to develop a similar device for adults known as NIVAC (noninvasive ventilatory assistance chamber). This device can be used for application of PEEP or CPAP.

Intermittent mandatory ventilation (IMV). Intermittent mandatory ventilation is a technique that was originally devised to wean patients from mechanical ventilation. As the term implies, the ventilation is intermittent yet mandatory. With this technique a number of breaths per minute are spontaneous and a number are delivered by the ventilator at a set tidal volume and rate each minute. This allows the patient to reeducate and strengthen his respiratory muscles during spontaneous ventilation and yet eases the work of breathing and ensures some good deep breaths as well. There is still some controversy about IMV because it is a relatively new technique. Certain criteria are to be met in most facilities before IMV is initiated.

Intermittent demand ventilation (IDV). Intermittent demand ventilation is a newer technique designed to augment ventilation by mechanically delivering intermittent positive pressure breaths on demand and *in phase* with a patient's own breathing pattern. The advantage of IDV over the use of IMV in the critically ill is that the former enhances spontaneous respiration, with a minimal elevation of intrathoracic pressure. Because of this, IDV is of particular value to patients with cardiovascular instability.

Drug therapy

A comprehensive guide to the drugs used in the treatment of respiratory failure is far beyond the scope of this text. A selection of those drugs most commonly used in the management of respiratory failure will be presented.

Drugs used in the treatment of infection. Infection is often a predisposing factor in respiratory failure, particularly in patients with chronic obstructive pulmonary disease. During the course of treatment of respiratory failure, infection may enter the body from several sources, such as a tracheostomy, an endotracheal tube, contaminated aerosol equipment, a urinary catheter, or at the site of an intravenous or arterial cannula. The choice of agent in treatment will depend on isolation of the offending pathogen. When clinical criteria indicate a respiratory infection, however, treatment is usually commenced pending specific bacteriologic diagnosis. A gram-stained sputum smear is used in these instances to aid in the selection of a suitable antibiotic. Drugs of choice in the treatment of respiratory infection may include the following.

Ampicillin. Ampicillin is a semisynthetic compound that has a broad spectrum of effectiveness. It is particularly effective in treatment of infections caused by *Hemophilus influenzae* and *Streptococcus viridans.* The dosage is usually 2 to 4 grams (Gm) daily, administered in four equal does, every 6 hours. Preparations of ampicillin are available for oral use as 250 or 500 mg capsules and for parenteral use as the sodium salt in vials containing 0.125, 0.25, 0.5, or 1 Gm.

Penicillin. Although one of the older antibiotics, penicillin is still the antibiotic of choice in the treatment of infections caused by the pneumococcus. The exception is the patient known to be allergic to the drug. Preparations of the penicillin most commonly used in the treatment of pneumococcal pneumonia are *penicillin G*, administered in doses of 500,000 to 1 million units every 6 hours given intramuscularly, or *procaine penicillin G*, administered as a single daily intramuscular injection in a dose of 600,000 units with or without the addition of 300,000 units of penicillin G.

Since *Hemophilus influenzae* or *Diplococcus pneumoniae* are the most common causative organisms in acute respiratory infections in patients with obstructive pulmonary disease, ampicillin and penicillin are often the drugs of choice to treat these infections.

Oxacillin (Prostaphlin). Oxacillin is a semisynthetic penicillin that is effective in treatment of penicillinase-producing staphylococci. It is also effective against susceptible pneumococci and streptococci. Preparations of oxacillin are available as sodium oxacillin for oral use in capsules containing 125, 250, or 500 mg. It is also available as sodium oxacillin for injection and may be given in doses of 2 to 4 Gm daily, intramuscularly or intravenously in four equal doses.

Side effects of the penicillins include hypersensitivity reactions, skin rashes, and eosinophilia.

Cephalothin (Keflin). Cephalothin is a derivative of cephalosporin C, one of a group of drugs known as the *cephalosporins.* It is active against a wide group of both gram-positive and gram-negative microorganisms and is particularly effective in infections produced by *Staphylococcus aureus, Streptococcus pyogenes,* and *Diplococcus pneumoniae.* Cephalothin is not suitable for oral use but can be used intramuscularly or intravenously. It is available in 10 ml rubber-stoppered vials containing 1 to 4 Gm. The dose administered varies with the degree of infection. In mild infections

1 Gm every 6 hours is usually adequate; however, for severe infections 1 Gm may be given every 2 hours. When the drug is given intravenously, 1 Gm should be dissolved in 20 to 30 ml of isotonic sodium chloride solution and infused over a period of 20 to 30 minutes. Another cephalosporin derivative in use is cephaloridine (Loridine).

Side effects that may result from cephalothin administration include pain, induration, sterile abscess, or tissue slough at the site of intramuscular injection. Phlebitis or thrombophlebitis is frequently associated with intravenous infusion of cephalothin. Hypersensitivity reactions may manifest themselves in the form of rashes, serum sickness, or anaphylaxis.

Other cephalosporins used include cephapirin (Cefadyl) for intravenous use in doses of 8 to 12 Gm per day; cefazolin (Ancef, Kefzol) for intramuscular use in doses of 1 to 6 Gm a day; and cephradine (Anspor, Velosef) for oral use in doses of 250 mg to 1 Gm every 6 hours.

Gentamicin sulfate (Garamycin sulfate). Gentamicin is a broad-spectrum antibiotic of the aminoglycoside group that is mainly effective in treating gram-negative microbacterial infections, particularly those caused by *Pseudomonas aeruginosa,* *Aerobacter,* and *Klebsiella.* Gentamicin is available in 2 ml vials containing a sterile solution of 40 mg/ml. The recommended dose is 3 to 5 mg/kg of body weight, given either every 8 hours or every 6 hours intramuscularly or intravenously. Pseudomonal infections are of major concern because they are difficult to treat and can spread rapidly. In certain instances more stubborn infections have been treated effectively by the use of a combination of gentamicin and carbenicillin disodium (Pyopen).

Side effects from gentamicin include nausea and vomiting, headache, transient proteinuria, transient macular skin eruptions, and, most important, involvement of the 8th cranial nerve. Impairment of vestibular and auditory function may be severe, and the incidence of these effects is increased in patients with renal insufficiency. Patients receiving gentamicin therapy should have their vestibular and auditory function checked frequently, and should be closely watched for changes in renal function. It is thought that cephalosporins and diuretics may markedly potentiate gentamicin nephrotoxicity. The drug should be discontinued if impairment is present.

Tobramycin (Nebcin). Tobramycin is a broad-spectrum antibiotic that is primarily used in treatment of gram-negative bacteria. Its action is similar to that of gentamicin, but studies suggest it is more effective in the treatment of *Pseudomonas aeruginosa* than is gentamicin. Tobramycin is available in 20 mg and 80 mg ampules and 60 mg and 80 mg disposable syringes. The recommended dose for patients with normal renal function is 3 to 4 mg/kg of body wieght daily intramuscularly or administered intravenously in 50 to 100 ml of diluent over a period of 20 to 60 minutes.

Side effects from tobramycin include impairment of auditory function, nephrotoxicity, thrombocytopenia, fever, urticaria, vomiting, headache, and lethargy. It is suggested that blood levels of tobramycin be monitored when used concurrently with carbenicillin, since tobramycin may be inactivated.

Drugs used in liquefaction of secretions. The presence of purulent, inspissated secretions is not uncommon in patients in respiratory failure who have respiratory infections. Many preparations are available to reduce the viscosity of sputum. Some of these include proteolytic enzymes, such as trypsin or pancreatic dornase, and acetylcysteine. These preparations are commonly grouped together as *mucolytic* agents, although the detergents liquefy sputum only by dilution, and the proteolytic enzymes function in the breakdown of sputum high in protein (purulent). There is some question as to whether mucolytic agents are more effective clinically than a 2% to 5% saline solution.

Acetylcysteine. Acetylcysteine (Mucomyst) is a sulfhydryl compound that liquefies mucus and DNA (the component of pus responsible for its viscosity) through the process of mucolysis. Liquefaction is apparent within 1 minute following administration, and a maximum effect occurs in 5 to 10 minutes. Acetylcysteine is available as a 20% sterile solution and is administered in a concentration of either 10% or 20% by a hand nebulizer or aerosol mask, by direct instillation via an endotracheal tube or tracheostomy, and by positive-pressure breathing apparatus. There is usually no set dosage schedule for the administration of acetylcysteine.

Side effects include bronchospasm and a burning sensation in the upper respiratory tract. The most common complaint from patients, however, is the odor of acetylcysteine, which is similar to rotten eggs.

Drugs used to relieve bronchospasm. An important part of management of many patients in respiratory failure is the relief of airways obstruction caused by bronchospasm. Bronchodilators are important drugs used in the relief of bronchospasm and are an integral part of basic bronchial hygiene. The two groups are the sympathomimetic drugs and the xanthines.

SYMPATHOMIMETIC DRUGS. A sympathomimetic drug is one that simulates the action of the sympathetic nervous system. The name was derived when a number of synthetic amines were studied and their pharmacologic activity was compared with the hormone epinephrine. Because of their chemical structure, certain sympathomimetics are termed *catecholamines,* which include norepinephrine, epinephrine, and isoproterenol.

The nurse will recall that there are three types of adrenergic receptors: alpha, beta-1, and beta-2. Norepinephrine stimulates alpha receptors predominantly, isoproterenol stimulates both beta receptors, and epinephrine stimulates all three receptors. The action of the catecholamines on beta-2 receptors is neurohumoral, with the conversion of adenosine triphosphate (ATP) to cyclic 3'-5'-adenosine monophosphate (cyclic AMP). (See Chapter 6.)

Epinephrine (Adrenalin). Epinephrine is a powerful bronchodilator because it (1) relaxes bronchial muscle and (2) is a physiologic antagonist to certain agents that constrict bronchial muscle (for example, histamine in bronchial asthma). Stimulation of beta-2 receptors results in bronchodilatation; stimulation, however, of beta-1 receptors in the myocardium makes epinephrine a powerful cardiac stimulant. The action of epinephrine on the alpha receptors relieves congestion of the bronchial mucosa, which is of a particular benefit to the patient with bronchial asthma in whom the condition is pronounced. Epinephrine is available as an injection, as a solution for inhalation by aerosol, or as a topical solution. In treatment of respiratory distress caused by bronchospasm, it is given in doses of 0.1 to 0.5 mg subcutaneously.

Side effects from epinephrine are many. It is highly toxic, which somewhat limits its use. Some of the effects include a feeling of fear, anxiety, tension, and restlessness. These are highly undesirable in patients who are already anxious. Ventricular arrhythmias may also occur.

Isoproterenol (Isuprel). Isoproterenol gives powerful beta-2 stimulation and therefore relaxes smooth muscle of the bronchial tree, thus acting as a bronchodilator. It is widely used in aerosol therapy, both in hospital practice and in treatment at home. The strong beta-1 stimulation of isoproterenol is responsible for the side effects presented later. Isoproterenol is available as isoproterenol hydrochloride inhalation in aerosol form and in solution. Aqueous solutions are available in concentrations of 1:100 and 1:200. They are usually administered in the 1:200 strength by hand nebulizer or a nebulizer in conjunction with IPPB. This may be on a 4-hourly schedule or when required. Commercial aerosols, known as Medihaler-Iso and Isuprel Mistometer, are also available.

Side effects include palpitation, tachycardia, and flushing of the skin. These effects occur frequently after treatment with isoproterenol. In some instances, serious arrhythmias, anginal pain, nausea, dizziness, and weakness also occur. A patient receiving isoproterenol should always have the apical and radial pulses checked simultaneously before, during, and after therapy. Any irregularity should be noted and the raise in pulse rate recorded.

Isoetharine. Isoetharine is a strong beta-2 receptor stimulant with little beta-1 activity. It is used in conjunction with phenylephrine as *Bronkosol* in a metered aerosol. The action of Bronkosol is of longer duration than that of Isuprel but the onset of action is slower. When bronchospasm is severe, this is a disadvantage because patients need immediate relief. Isoetharine is also available as an oral preparation (Dilabron).

Side effects from isoetharine include tachycardia, headache, nausea, anxiety, and restlessness.

SELECTIVE BETA-2 STIMULANTS. Several drugs are now available for the relief of bronchospasm with selective beta-2 receptor stimulation. This is a highly desirable feature of a drug for the asthmatic patient because of the bronchodilating effect with less of the cardioexcitary effects of beta-1 stimulation.

Metaproterenol (Alupent or Metaprel) is available as a metered aerosol and as 20 mg tablets. The advantages of inhaled metaproterenol is its length of action: approximately 3 to 4 hours compared with 1 hour for Isuprel and 2 hours for Bronkosol.

Side effects with inhaled metaproterenol are relatively few but may include nervousness, tremor, nausea, and tachycardia. These side effects are severe when the drug is administered orally.

Terbutaline (Bricanyl) is available as an oral preparation in 2.5 to 5 mg tablets and also as an injectable in ampules with 1 mg/ml. The adult dosage is 1 tablet three times a day. The drug is long acting with bronchodilatation lasting up to 7 hours.

Side effects from terbutaline are nervousness, tremor, and palpitation.

Several selective beta-2 drugs already in use in Europe and Canada are now being tested in the United States. These include fenoterol (Berotec), salbutamol (Ventolin), and ritodrine (Premar).

THE XANTHINES. Caffeine, theophylline, and theobromine are known as the xanthines and are central nervous system stimulants. They also have several other important actions. They produce diuresis by their action on the kidney, they stimulate cardiac muscle, and most important to our interest, they relax smooth muscle, notably bronchial smooth muscle. The xanthines work as bronchodilators by increasing levels of cyclic AMP through inactivating phosphodiesterase, a substance that normally breaks down cyclic AMP.

Aminophylline. Aminophylline is derived from the compound theophylline and is most effective of the xanthines in relaxing the smooth muscles of the bronchi. Aminophylline is a most powerful bronchodilator. Action of the drug on the medulla also stimulates respiration by increasing the rate and depth of breathing. Aminophylline is used extensively in the treatment of bronchial asthma and is particularly valuable when attacks are prolonged. Preparations of aminophylline for intravenous injection are available in ampules containing 250 mg/10 ml and 500 mg/20 ml. Rectal suppositories are supplied in 125, 250, or 500 mg sizes, and tablets for oral administration are available in 100 or 200 mg sizes.

In the treatment of intractable bronchial asthma, an initial loading dose of 5 to 6 mg/kg of body weight is given by slow intravenous injection over 15 to 30 minutes and will generally give the patient prompt relief. Continued therapy is usually indicated and may be administered by continuous intravenous infusion or by the use of rectal suppositories.

Side effects include nausea, vomiting, restlessness, diaphoresis, and a fall in blood pressure. The fine line between safe levels of aminophylline makes it important to watch carefully for side effects, particularly during intravenous administration of the drug. If the drug is given too rapidly, the patient may have a cardiac arrest.

COMBINATION PREPARATIONS. Combination preparations of theophylline and its derivatives are too numerous to cover completely in this section, but some of the more popular drugs are presented in Table 11.

Drugs used specifically in the treatment of asthma often include not only those for the relief of bronchospasm but also corticosteroids: *disodium cromoglycate* or *cromolyn sodium (Intal, Aarane).* The role of cromolyn sodium is thought to be prophylactic by preventing mediator release from mast cells of histamine and slow-reacting substance of anaphylaxis. The use of cromolyn sodium has enabled some patients to reduce their dosage of corticosteroids and in some cases discontinue them altogether. Cromolyn sodium is available as a 20 mg capsule, which contains a powder that is inhaled with the use of a special inhaler. The patient should be properly instructed in use of the inhaler before treatment begins.

CORTICOSTEROIDS. Corticosteroids are used in the treatment of asthma either in

TABLE 11. Combination preparations of theophylline and its derivatives

Trade name	Generic name	Amount of drug in milligrams	Adult dose
Amesec	Aminophylline Ephedrine hydrochloride Amytal	130 25 25	1 to 5 capsules in 24-hour period
Aminodur Dura-Tabs	Aminophylline	300	1 to 2 tablets every 8 to 12 hours 30 minutes before eating
Bronkotabs	Theophylline Ephedrine Phenobarbital Glyceryl guaiacolate	100 24 8 100	1 tablet every 3 to 4 hours
Choledyl	Oxytriphylline	200—yellow tablet 100—red tablet 100—elixir	200 or 100 mg 4 times a day or 2 teaspoons 4 times a day
Marax	Theophylline Ephedrine Hydroxyzine	130 25 10	1 tablet 2 to 4 times a day
Quadrinal	Theophylline Ephedrine Phenobarbital Potassium iodide	130 24 24 320	1 tablet 3 to 4 times a day
Tedral	Theophylline Ephedrine Phenobarbital	130 25 8	1 to 2 tablets every 4 hours
Lufyllin	Dyphylline dihydroxypropyl Theophylline	200—tablet 100—elixir	1 tablet 3 to 4 times a day or 2 tablespoons

conjunction with other therapy to treat a severe attack or to maintain the unstable patient already receiving conventional therapy. In the acute phase high doses of corticosteroids may be needed, for example, 60 to 80 mg a day with gradual reduction of the dosage. Maintenance doses usually range from 2.5 to 20 mg a day, but are generally regulated using eosinophil counts as an indicator of the effectiveness of therapy.

Corticosteroid aerosols are being used with increasing frequency. *Beclomethasone dipropionate* is one such aerosol, which is believed can replace or reduce the dosage of systemic corticosteroids in some patients.

Drugs used to stimulate respiration. There are various schools of thought on the value of respiratory stimulants, but because they are used, the drugs commonly employed will be presented.

Ethamivan (Emivan). Ethamivan is a general central nervous system stimulant. It significantly increases respiratory tidal volume and also partially restores the sensitivity to carbon dioxide of the respiratory center. Ethamivan is available for intravenous injection in 2 and 10 ml ampules containing 50 mg/ml. Because of the short duration of the effects of the drug (10 to 30 minutes), it is usually administered as a continuous intravenous infusion, using 1 Gm in 250 ml of 5% dextrose delivered at a rate of 0.05 to 0.15 mg/kg of body weight. The patient's blood gases are monitored to ascertain the degree of reduction in arterial PCO_2 as an evaluation of the effectiveness of therapy.

Side effects from ethamivan include muscular twitching and seizures; the latter occur infrequently.

Nikethamide (Coramine). Nikethamide is a synthetic compound that stimulates the central nervous system. It has a strong stimulative action on a depressed respiratory center. Nikethamide increases the sensitivity of the respiratory center to carbon dioxide. The drug is usually administered by intermittent intravenous injection on a 2-hourly basis for six doses. Dosage of nikethamide is regulated by starting the patient with a small dose of 20 mg/kg of body weight, which is then increased to a level where the patient is arousable and the arterial PCO_2 is lowered.

Intravenous injection of nikethamide is followed by unpleasant *side effects*, which include sneezing, vomiting, facial irritation, and intense mental distress. When these effects occur, the patient becomes more alert and should be encouraged to clear secretions. Treatment is not continued for more than 12 hours because of the severe agitation and obvious distress of the patient. If effective reduction in arterial PCO_2 is not apparent after 12 hours, treatment is discontinued.

Doxapram hydrochloride (Dopram). Doxapram is one of the newer respiratory stimulants, and its site of action is thought to be direct stimulation of the carotid bodies. Doxapram is considered to be a little safer than other respiratory stimulants, but it is not without side effects. Doxapram is available for intravenous injection in 20 ml vials, and it may be administered as divided intravenous doses of 0.5 to 1.5 mg/kg.

Side effects include tachycardias, arrhythmias, sneezing, vomiting, itching, and tremors.

Drugs used in the treatment of acid-base disturbances. Correction of acid-base disturbances is a major element in the treatment of patients in respiratory failure. The respiratory stimulants previously discussed are used in the treatment of acid-base disturbances because of their effect on carbon dioxide elimination. Other drugs include buffering agents and carbonic anhydrase inhibitors.

Sodium bicarbonate ($NaHCO_3$). Sodium bicarbonate is an alkalizing agent that functions physiologically as an inorganic buffer. Sodium bicarbonate is used in the correction of metabolic acidosis to increase the level of bicarbonate in the blood, which then is available to combine with the excess hydrogen ions. The result is carbonic acid, which becomes dehydrated to $CO_2 + H_2O$, and the CO_2 is then excreted by way of the lungs. Sodium bicarbonate for injection is available in 50 ml ampules containing 7.5% and as a 5% solution in 500 ml intravenous bottles.

When treating metabolic acidosis resulting from the accumulation of lactic acid during cardiac arrest, large amounts of bicarbonate are required to correct the disturbance. Initially treatment is usually three to five 50 ml ampules (44 mEq) given rapidly by intravenous injection. From 200 to 800 mEq of sodium bicarbonate are often required to correct the acidosis, and 1 ampule may be given every 5 minutes until effective circulation is restored. Careful monitoring of arterial pH is used as a guide to sodium bicarbonate administration.

It should be remembered that the underlying cause of the acidosis must be treated and that the two dangers of sodium bicarbonate administration are excessive sodium or overdosage resulting in a metabolic alkalosis.

THAM. THAM is tris (hydroxymethyl) aminomethane, a buffer that has been used in the treatment of acute respiratory acidosis. THAM combines with carbon dioxide to form bicarbonate and thus restore pH. The value of the drug has been questioned, since its administration may result in depressed ventilation and apnea. Therefore equipment for mechanical ventilation should always be ready when the drug is used. Also the drug is not a substitute for restoration of adequate ventilation and appears to be of value only in short-term treatment where normal ventilation can be restored within a few hours (for example, in the treatment of acute respiratory acidosis associated with status asthmaticus). The drug is administered by intravenous infusion as a 0.3 molar solution in 2% sodium chloride at a rate of 300 ml/hr.

Acetazolamide (Diamox). The action of acetazolamide is to inhibit the enzyme carbonic anhydrase, which speeds the following chemical reaction within the erythrocyte:

$$CO_2 + H_2O \xrightleftharpoons[\text{}]{\text{Carbonic anhydrase}} H_2CO_3$$

Inhibition of carbonic anhydrase activity results in slowing CO_2 uptake from the tissues and CO_2 unloading in the lungs. Ventilation is usually improved accompanied by improved oxygenation of the blood. There has been some limited success using carbonic anhydrase inhibitors in patients with abnormally high levels of carbon dioxide in relationship to their ventilation. The action of the drug is slow and may persist for several days.

Hydration

Deviations from normal body fluid and electrolyte balance are commonly encountered in patients in respiratory failure. These deviations may result from inadequate fluid and dietary intake, diuretic therapy, acid-base irregularities, abnormal elimination (for example, vomiting), sweating, or abnormal renal function. Fluid excess or deficit is accompanied by changes in electrolytes, and these, combined with acid-base imbalances occurring in the patient with respiratory failure, may be extremely dangerous.

A patient is evaluated in terms of his fluid and electrolyte status by careful measurement and assessment of total daily fluid intake and output, daily weights, examination of the skin and mucous membranes, consistency of pulmonary secretions, and serum electrolyte studies. Dehydration is reflected by a dry, warm skin with loss of elastic tone. The tongue may be enlarged and dry, and when dehydration is severe, the eyes are sunken. Adequate systemic hydration is as necessary to keeping pulmonary secretions thin as is humidification of the inspired air, and this factor should be considered if a patient's sputum becomes thickened. A sudden loss of weight may reflect excessive fluid loss; before treatment is initiated in this instance, other data and a repeat weight should be obtained.

Laboratory findings in the dehydrated patient include an acute increase in hematocrit because of hemoconcentration. This must be differentiated from the rise in hematocrit occurring in patients with chronic lung disease. Urinalysis of the dehydrated patient will reflect an increase in specific gravity because of increase in urine concentration.

Overhydration is also a danger to the patient in respiratory failure because of the complications of hypervolemia or pulmonary edema. Predisposing factors to hypervolemia, such as prolonged steroid therapy or congestive heart failure, may be present in the patient with chronic lung disease and are an additional danger if excess fluid is administered.

Clinical findings include pitting edema of the skin, moist rales heard throughout the lungs (which may increase with the manifestation of pulmonary edema), a sudden weight gain, and venous engorgement. Excess fluid may be administered to the patient intravenously or orally. It is important that all intake, such as ice chips, fluids used to flush intravenous and intra-arterial catheters, and all other parenteral and oral fluids, be measured accurately. Ultrasonic nebulizers have been known to overhydrate a patient, and this possibility must be considered, particularly in patients with renal or cardiac conditions who are on strict fluid balance.

Serum electrolyte studies of the important cations (sodium [Na], potassium [K], calcium [Ca]) and the anions (chlorides [Cl], phosphates, sulfates, and protein) are important not only in evaluating the degree of hydration but also as clues to acid-base disturbances because of changes in cation-anion balances. Two important elements in a patient's electrolyte and hydration status are the amount of water lost through respiration and the amount of water and electrolytes lost through sweating. Water is lost through the lungs on an average of 600 to 1,000 ml daily; this may be considerably increased or decreased in the patient in respiratory failure. Normal body sweat is a hypotonic solution containing sodium, potassium, and chloride. A febrile patient may lose a considerable amount of fluid and electrolytes through the skin as sweat. It is important to remember that only the extracellular electrolytes are being measured, and these may not always reflect what is happening within the cells.

Removal of secretions

A major problem occurring in the patient in respiratory failure is the collection of secretions. In some patients, particularly those with chronic obstructive lung disease, an underlying infection may result in the accumulation of copious amounts of purulent, inspissated secretions. When secretions collect in the respiratory tract, airways obstruction is increased and atelectasis often occurs beyond the obstruction. This results in maldistribution of ventilation with respect to blood flow and an increased physiologic shunt.

Mobilization of microsecretions. Two types of pulmonary secretions have been mentioned (Chapter 7), those that reside in the larger airways (macrosecretions) and those that reside in the smaller airways (microsecretions). Techniques such as postural drainage and percussion are not effective in the mobilization of microsecretions, so additional techniques of physiotherapy are employed. These involve hyperinflation of the lung, manual compression, and special coughing techniques.

The procedure is explained to the patient, and then he is postured so that once the microsecretions are dislodged, special coughing techniques will transfer them to the major airways where they can be removed by gravity drainage, suctioning, or normal coughing. Two people, usually a physiotherapist and a nurse or physician, are required to conduct the procedure. First the patient's lungs are hyperinflated by IPPB or a hand inflation unit to introduce air distal to the secretions. Then during expiration the therapist applies chest-wall compression intermittently, which literally squeezes out the air in short, rapid bursts and dislodges secretions. This method of artificial coughing is most effective in prevention and treatment of atelectasis.

Following hyperinflation of the lungs, a patient can also be encouraged to take a series of short coughs with his mouth and glottis open; these are known as "huff coughs," because of the sound made as the patient performs the technique. This technique has two important advantages: (1) it reduces pain from coughing because there is no great increase in intrapulmonic and abdominal pressure; and (2) it prevents the airways collapse that occurs with rapid expiration in patients with chronic obstructive pulmonary disease.

Some patients require more than normal physiotherapy techniques to stimulate an effective cough or to mobilize or remove microsecretions. Methods that can be used for these purposes include cricothyroid cannulation to induce cough, special physiotherapy techniques, and fiberoptic bronchoscopy for removal of secretions.

Cricothyroid cannulation. An effective method used to induce cough is cricothyroid cannulation. Following surgical cleansing of the neck and infiltration of the skin with local anesthetic, a small polyethylene catheter is introduced over a needle into the trachea through the cricothyroid membrane.

The position of the catheter is checked by instilling 2 to 5 ml of normal saline through it into the trachea; the patient's response will be a deep cough when the catheter is well placed. An antibacterial ointment is applied at the site of insertion on a small dressing, and the catheter is taped securely in place. Saline is then instilled into the catheter when necessary to stimulate cough.

Flexible fiberoptic bronchoscopy (FFB). When secretions cannot be removed employing any of the methods previously described, FFB may be indicated. This technique is of particular value when atelectasis is present due to retained secretions, which are usually thick, tenacious mucus plugs. It can also be used in the diagnosis and control of hemoptysis, as a diagnostic procedure for lesions in the airways, and as an aid to difficult intubation.

The procedure is explained to the patient, and a signed permit is obtained if possible. An anxious patient may require premedication or titrated sedation (usually diazepam) during the procedure. Local anesthesia of 2 to 3 ml of 1% Xylocaine is frequently injected transtracheally through the cricoid membrane. Topical anesthesia of viscous Xylocaine is instilled into the selected nasal passage. Additional anesthesia is then applied to the vocal chords and pharynx as the bronchoscope is inserted.

Because of its length (180 cm), the FFB can be passed down into the subsegmental bronchi. During passage of the fiberoptic bronchoscope, the airways are carefully inspected for lesions of any kind. Secretions are removed by way of the suction channel of the FFB following instillation of sterile normal saline. At this time aspirated secretions can be obtained for culture.

Fiberoptic bronchoscopy can be used during mechanical ventilation by using special adaptors for the equipment without interrupting mechanical ventilation.

Parameters that are usually monitored with fiberoptic bronchoscopy include electrocardiogram; intratracheal pressure; arterial blood gases before, during, and after the procedure; inspired oxygen concentration, which is usually kept at 60% during the procedure; and chest x-ray examination to check for possible pneumothorax.

Prevention of infection

In patients with chronic obstructive pulmonary disease, an acute infection is often the predisposing factor that tilts the delicate balance of already impaired gas exchange into respiratory failure. Nurses probably more than any other members of the health team are in a position to guard this group of patients from further infection and to prevent infection from occurring among the noninfected patients in respiratory failure. This is not always an easy task because it means not only meticulous nursing but seeing that equipment is frequently sterilized and that other health team members also apply stringent standards to prevent infection.

Elements that predispose infection. Sterility of the lower respiratory tract is normally maintained by mucociliary function, alveolar macrophages, pulmonary lymphatics, and the normal cough (Chapter 1). Periodic hyperinflation of the lungs, which occurs with the normal sigh, also contributes to healthy alveoli by preventing atelectasis and by stimulating surfactant production. Usually these mechanisms are depressed or interrupted in patients in respiratory failure because of either the underlying condition or necessary elements of management, such as tracheostomy, endotracheal intubation, oxygen therapy, and mechanical ventilation. Therefore the patients' defenses are reduced against the invasion and proliferation of bacteria.

Sources of infection. The most common sources from which bacteria enter the respiratory tract of the hospitalized patient are contaminated respiratory therapy equipment (aerosols and humidification equipment in particular), careless suctioning techniques, and solutions standing in open containers. It should be kept in mind that a hospital environment is a constant threat to the debilitated patient in terms of infection. Most hospitals have their own particular strain of *Staphylococcus,* and it has been estimated that 90% of infections due to staphylococci are caused by the resident hospital strain. Cross-infection is a well-known and documented problem; nonetheless, it is still most serious and something that health team members can do much to prevent.

Patients requiring intensive respiratory care are subject to bacterial invasion from many other sources. These include any site of cannulation—intravenous, intra-arterial, or cricothyroid or by way of a catheter in the urinary bladder.

Recognition of infection. The seriousness of even a minor infection should never be underestimated. It gives an already ill patient one more battle to fight. Early recognition of an infection means early treatment and generally more effective control. Fever and the presence of purulent sputum are clear indications of respiratory tract infection and warrant immediate treatment. Frequent laboratory examination of pulmonary secretions facilitates the early detection of respiratory infection and isolation of the causative microorganism. It is recommended that deep tracheal aspirate be obtained from tracheostomized or intubated patients. The aspirate should be collected in a sterile mucus trap and sent for sputum culture and sensitivity every other day.

Methods of prevention. To prevent infection in the respiratory patient, the following guidelines should be observed:

1. Meticulously remove all secretions. Use sterile suction catheters, sterile gloves, and so on one time only.

2. Treat tracheostomies as a surgical wound, and always use aseptic techniques when handling the tracheostomy or any equipment that comes into contact with it.

3. See that all wet parts (tubing, valves, humidifiers, nebulizers) of respiratory therapy are replaced with sterile parts at least every 12 hours and preferably during each shift.

4. Perform routine chest physiotherapy to prevent pooling of secretions and atelectasis, both of which predispose to infection.

5. Change dressings frequently at all sites of cannulation, using a suitable antibiotic ointment.

6. Use isolation precautions and facilities to prevent cross-infection.

7. Pay attention to general patient care, such as personal hygiene, nutrition, and hydration requirements, to increase the patient's own natural defenses against infection.

Prevention of infection is far better than cure. A patient receiving antibiotic therapy is by no means protected from the invasion of bacteria; this in fact may predispose a superinfection by a more virulent microorganism.

Rehabilitation

An important element when caring for the patient in respiratory failure is rehabilitation, which is a continuous process beginning the moment a patient is hospitalized and continuing long after discharge in many instances. There are two main approaches to rehabilitation, but with considerable overlap: physical and psychosocial. The nurse plays an important role in the delivery of these aspects of health care, which for clarity will be discussed separately.

Physical rehabilitation. Adequate nutrition and hydration are important aspects of rehabilitation and, unless contraindicated, the nurse should encourage patients to take all the nourishment allowed by mouth. The oral route is the most satisfactory way of supplying a patient with sufficient calories and should not be neglected because a patient requires complete assistance with feeding or constant supervision during a meal.

Physiotherapy is not only essential to the prevention and treatment of respiratory complications but also in preventing and treating loss of musculoskeletal integrity. Such programs include simple range-of-motion exercises and increasing patient activity levels from "dangling" to sitting out of bed in a chair to ambulation. For patients who have suffered injury from automobile accidents or cerebrovascular accident, physiotherapy programs are often extensive in order to restore body function. Oxygen-assisted ambulation is often required in patients with chronic lung disease and in patients who are being "weaned" from mechanical ventilation.

Patients with respiratory difficulties frequently have to work hard in order to breathe, and this fact should be kept in mind when any physical exercise is performed by the patient. The patient must be allowed to take his time and to rest when necessary. If an exercise program is too exhausting, the patient will not tolerate it well. Instead of feeling encouraged by progress, he will suffer the distress of a setback, which may lead him to refuse further exercise.

Psychosocial rehabilitation. Every member of the health team who has any patient contact is in a position to aid intermittently in a patient's psychosocial rehabilitation. The nurse at the bedside is, however, in this position constantly. A necessary ingredient in this aspect of care is communication, a sharing of information between physicians, nurses, therapists, and patients and their families, which will benefit total patient care and strengthen the bond between health team members.

Many patients in respiratory failure find themselves in an intensive respiratory care unit quite suddenly. For example, a victim of an automobile accident is on the road one minute and in bed with tubes entering every available orifice the next. Usually such patients will have had lapses of consciousness caused either by trauma or sedation. On awakening they will have dozens of questions and yet be unable to verbalize them because of endotracheal intubation or tracheostomy.

Psychosocial rehabilitation begins at once. Tell the patient where he is and why he is there. Explain that he will be unable to speak for a little while and show him a method of nonverbal communication. Introduce yourself. Show the patient where the clock and calendar are so he knows what time it is and what day it is. Find out whether he normally requires glasses to see his surroundings. Reassure the patient that he will not be left alone and explain the purpose of the various pieces of equipment. As you conduct nursing procedures, explain them to your patient while remembering that he is in a totally foreign environment and that much medical jargon sounds like a different language to him.

Unless oriented through special hospital programs, the family members entering a critical care area for the first time are usually horrified by what they see. It is up to the nursing staff to put the patient's family at ease in this situation, answering questions where possible, orienting them to the hospital facilities, and finding the patient's physician to speak with the family when necessary.

A patient in a busy hospital setting must be protected from his environment. Nurses can do this by keeping noise at a minimum and allowing the patient to rest whenever possible between busy treatment schedules and frequent monitoring of vital signs. Sleep deprivation and sensory overstimulation not infrequently occur in patients undergoing intensive care. This is not conducive to either psychosocial rehabilitation or physical rehabilitation.

A major consideration in psychosocial rehabilitation is the loss of personal dignity and self-esteem a patient may feel. Many things about himself may frustrate and disgust him—dependence on others and machines for survival, that he is no longer a wage earner, the question of how his family is managing, and the need of assistance with his eliminations. His own secretions may disgust and embarrass him. Looming large in the patient's mind is also the fear of death. A patient once told me that each time the nurses disconnected him from a ventilator to remove secretions he was sure that they would forget to put him back and that he would die. In that particular patient this led to severe sleep deprivation and much mental suffering. A nurse's awareness and sensitivity to patient needs will provide a firm foundation for alleviating many of the fears and anxieties the hospitalized patient experiences.

The goals of physical and psychosocial rehabilitation are to prepare the patient for transfer from the critical care setting as soon as his condition will allow, with the constant encouragement that one day the patient will leave the hospital. This requires total communication between all members of the health team. On an intensive respiratory care unit this means joint patient conferences between *all* team members: nurses, physicians, physiotherapists, respiratory therapists, and psychiatric social workers. Everyone has something to contribute.

REFERENCES

Bendixen, H. H., Egbert, L. D., Headly-Whyte, J., Laver, M. B., and Pontoppidan, H.: Respiratory care, St. Louis, 1965, The C. V. Mosby Co.

Caroll, R. G., and Grenvik, A.: Proper use of large diameter residual volume cuffs, Crit. Care Med. 1:153, 1973.

Cassem, N. H., and Hackett, T. P.: Stress on the nurse and therapist in the intensive-care unit and the coronary-care unit, Heart Lung 4:252-259, 1975.

Egan, D. F.: Fundamentals of respiratory therapy, ed. 2, St. Louis, 1973, The C. V. Mosby Co.

Fisher, E. J.: Antimicrobial therapy: some guidelines, Heart Lung 5:437-442, 1976.

Goodman, L. S., and Gilman, A., editors: The pharmacological basis of therapeutics, ed. 5, New York, 1975, The Macmillan Co.

Hargreaves, A. G.: Emotional problems of patients with respiratory diseases, Nurs. Clin. North Am. 3:479-488, 1968.

Katz, N. M., Agle, D. P., DePalma, R. G., and DeCossee, J. J.: Delirium in surgical patients under intensive care, utility of mental status examination, Arch. Surg. 104:310-313, 1972.

King, K., Mandava, B., and Kamen, J. M.: Tracheal tube cuffs and tracheal dilatation, Chest 67:458-462, 1975.

Lindholm, C. E., Ollman, B., Snyder, J., Millen,

E., and Grenvik, A.: Flexible fiberoptic bronchoscopy in critical care medicine: diagnosis,
therapy and complications, Crit. Care Med.
2:250-262, 1974.

Pontoppidan, H., Geffin, B., and Lowenstein, E.:
Acute respiratory failure in the adult (in three
parts), N. Engl. J. Med. **287:**690-698, 743-752,
799-806, 1972.

Selecky, P. A.: Tracheostomy: a review of present
day indications, complications, and care, Heart
Lung **3:**272-283, 1974.

Shapiro, B. A., Harrison, R. A., Walton, J. R.,
and Davidson, R.: Intermittent demand ventilation (IDV): a new technique for supporting
ventilation in critically ill patients, Respir.
Care **21:**521-525, 1976.

Sugerman, H. J., Rogers, R. M., and Miller, L. D.:
Positive end expiratory pressure (PEEP): indications and physiologic considerations, Chest **62**
(supp.):86S-94S, 1972.

Tyler, M. L.: Artificial airway—suctioning, tubes
and cuffs weaning and extubation, Nursing
73(2):21-36, 1973.

Wanner, A., Landa, J. F., Nieman, R. E., Ver-
aina, J., and Delgado, I.: Bedside broncho-
fiberoscopy for atelectasis and lung abscess,
J.A.M.A. **224:**1281-1283, 1973.

Wilson, R. F., and Sibbald, W. J.: Acute respiratory failure, Crit. Care Med. **4:**79-89, 1976.

10 / INTENSIVE RESPIRATORY CARE IN SPECIFIC CONDITIONS

Recognition by hospital administrators of the necessity for respiratory intensive care units, staffed by well-trained health care teams, has contributed greatly to the survival of patients in respiratory failure. Although patients with a wide variety of conditions may require intensive respiratory care, certain specific conditions will be given special attention in this chapter.

EMERGENCY RESUSCITATION

Respiratory or cardiac arrest requires immediate effective resuscitative measures if the patient is to be saved from death or irreversible brain damage. Initially the arrest may be either respiratory or cardiac, but in either situation one will follow the other within minutes or less.

Management of respiratory arrest

In hospital practice complete cessation of breathing most commonly occurs following cardiac arrest. It may also occur following blockage of the upper airway or tube blockage by a foreign body or secretions, after drug overdosage, cerebrovascular accident, drowning, or electrocution. Accidents with mechanical ventilatory equipment in the already apneic patient will also result in respiratory arrest. There is no time to lose in attempting to reverse the process. The American Heart Association Committee on Cardiopulmonary Resuscitation (CPR) and Emergency Cardiac Care (ECC) have attempted to standardize resuscitation techniques by presenting recommendations for procedure and training. The order of management for respiratory arrest or cardiac arrest presented here includes those guidelines for basic life support (witnessed cardiac arrest) and advanced life support (monitored patient). The ABCs of CPR are A, airway; B, breathing; and C, circulation.

1. Call for help
2. Establish airway patency (A): hyperextend the neck and lift the jaw forward
3. Restore breathing (ventilation) (B) using
   a. Mouth-to-mouth ventilation
   b. Ventilation bag with mask
   c. Intubation and mechanical ventilation

4. Restore circulation *(C)* using
   a. External cardiac compression
   b. Defibrillation

Airway patency. Before any resuscitative procedure can be effective, an open airway must be established. Any obvious secretions should be removed from the oropharynx (vomit, mucus) by suction, if available, or by hand using a gauze sponge around the fingers to scoop out debris or dentures. If an endotracheal or tracheostomy tube is in situ, tube and cuff patency must be checked. To clear the tongue from the back of the throat and open the upper airway, the patient's neck should be hyperextended and the head tilted as far back as possible. This is accomplished by first removing the bed pillow, then lifting the neck with one hand and maximally tilting the head backward with the other. A thick roll of towels or sheets placed beneath the shoulders of the patient will help to maintain this position. The nurse's hands will then be free to hold the jaw forward and apply artificial ventilation (Fig. 10-1, *D*).

Ventilation and oxygenation. Once the airway is open with correct positioning of the neck and head, the patient can be ventilated. This may be achieved by using expired air ventilation, a mask with self-inflating bag, or intubation and mechanical ventilation.

Expired air ventilation should be initiated immediately if no other equipment is available. This may be mouth-to-mouth or mouth-to-nose resuscitation and should be carried out by the nurse in the following way:

1. Clear the patient's airway and position the patient's head and neck as described earlier. To use the mouth-to-mouth method occlude the patient's nostrils with the thumb and forefinger of one hand, while at the same time applying pressure to the patient's forehead to maintain the backward tilt.

2. Take in a deep breath; place your mouth completely over the patient's mouth and exhale as forcibly and evenly as possible, watching through the corner of your eye for inflation of the patient's chest.

3. Remove your mouth and passive exhalation follows; repeat the procedure every 5 seconds. The initial procedure, however, should be four full quick breaths.

Effectiveness of mouth-to-mouth ventilation can be ascertained by the rise and fall of the patient's chest, the degree of resistance and compliance of the patient's lungs felt in your own airway as you inflate them, and the escape of air during passive exhalation.

Many types of airways and S-tubes are available to use in conjunction with mouth-to-mouth resuscitation. They usually are of plastic or heavy-duty rubber and divided by a flange that permits one end of the tube to be inserted over the tongue in the patient's mouth. A seal is formed by the flange around the patient's lips. The other end of the tube is used by the operator to inflate the lungs. An S-tube may be used in the infected patient.

Another aid to establishing ventilation in CPR is the use of the esophageal obturator. This is designed as a combination cuffed endotracheal tube and mask with the addition of a soft plastic obturator located in the distal end of the tube and a series of holes (to allow the passage of air) in the upper third of the tube. The tube is inserted into the esophagus and the cuff inflated to seal off the esophagus; then the patient is ventilated, either mouth-to-tube with a bag and tube or with a mechanical ventilator. The port on the mask piece provides attachment for the equipment used, and the air delivered enters the trachea via the openings in the tube.

The esophageal obturator has been found to be of particular value in transporting the critically injured patient because it can be inserted without direct visualization and can be used in circumstances where the injured person is difficult to reach for mouth-to-mouth ventilation; for example, the victim of an automobile accident trapped under the car.

Training is required in the insertion of the esophageal obturator, but it is a simpler technique than endotracheal intubation. Complications may arise by damage to the oropharynx or the esophagus when an untrained person uses the tube.

The disadvantage of the esophageal airway is that the patient may vomit as the tube

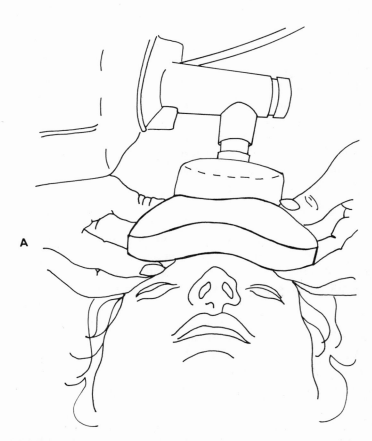

A

FIG. 10-1. A, Correct technique for holding a ventilation bag and mask prior to application. Note that the mask is being stretched.

is inserted and frequently vomits when the tube is removed. Precautions should therefore be taken to prevent aspirtion of gastric contents.

During any procedure for emergency respiratory resuscitation, the patient's pulses are palpated to make sure circulation is being maintained.

A ventilation bag with mask is widely used in emergency resuscitation. The equipment usually consists of a self-inflating bag, a nonreturn valve (to prevent re-breathing), anesthetic-type masks of various sizes, suitable adaptors for use with endo-tracheal and tracheostomy tubes, and an inlet for oxygen delivery. It is most desirable that nurses know to how to use the self-inflating bag and mask. Fig. 10-1 illustrates the techniques of mask application and operation. Before starting bag and mask resus-citation, an open airway must be established and the patient's neck and head placed in the correct position; the nurse should then proceed in the following order:

1. Stand behind the patient's head. This involves either removing the headboard from the bed or moving the patient partially across the bed, bringing his head closer to the edge. Insert an oral airway to maintain airway patency.

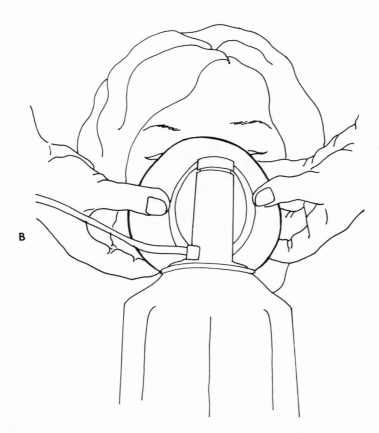

B

FIG. 10-1, cont'd. B, The stretched mask is positioned on the patient's face. As the mask resumes its original shape, the patient's skin is pulled inward.   *Continued.*

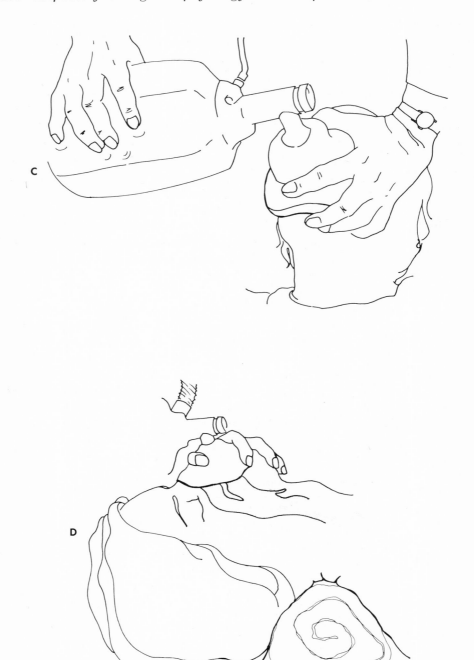

FIG. 10-1, cont'd. C, Ventilation bag and mask in use. Note position of thumb and forefinger around the mask. Remaining fingers maintain hyperextension of the head and support the jaw. **D,** Side view of ventilation bag and mask application illustrates the open airway obtained by hyperextension of the head.

2. Hold the mask in both hands between the thumbs and forefingers and apply a pulling maneuver to the edges of the mask as you tightly position the mask over the patient's nose and mouth. The patient's skin will be gathered into the mask as the mask resumes its normal position, providing a tight seal (Fig. 10-1, *A* and *B*).

3. Hold the mask firmly in place with one hand; use the same hand to maintain the head tilt and hyperextension of the neck and to support the jaw. Use your free hand to squeeze the bag, which forces air into the patient's lungs (Fig. 10-1, *C* and *D*).

4. When ventilation is adequate, the chest should rise and fall; you should feel resistance of the bag during inflation and should hear air escape during exhalation. Airways obstruction and changes in lung compliance will be reflected as increased resistance of the bag as you compress it. A quick check for airway patency and reapplication of the mask are necessary if this occurs.

With each complete squeeze of the bag a volume of approximately 1,000 to 1,400 ml (stroke volume) will be delivered to a patient, depending on the make of the bag. Oxygen concentrations of up to 60% can be achieved with some ventilating bags, and the concentration usually depends on the rate of oxygen flow.

Investigations into the efficiency of resuscitator bags and other hand-operated emergency ventilation devices have shown that certain makes of ventilating bags are superior in many ways to others. One of these is the Laerdal bag (Resusci folding bag), model RFB-11, which has a transparent bag and mask that allows direct visualization of the oropharynx; secretions can be spotted immediately. It also has a reservoir tube, which maintains a high concentration of inspired oxygen at rates of flow of 10 liters/min. Models of Air Shields ("AMBU" with E-2 valve) and the Puritan PMR are also recommended. Certain devices were found to be dangerous and are in the process of being withdrawn. These are Clar Aire bag and Res-Q-Air bag.

Intubation and mechanical ventilation. Inadequacy of ventilation by bag and mask is marked by increased resistance to chest inflation, poor chest movement, and rapidly increasing gastric distention. In these circumstances or when it is anticipated that mechanical support to ventilation will be needed for some time (for example, in drug overdosage or failure to establish adequate ventilation and oxygenation in a cardiac arrest), endotracheal intubation and mechanical ventilation are usually instituted. Any type of assisted ventilatory technique should be followed as early as possible by the insertion of a nasogastric tube to relieve distention. Insertion of this tube will help to prevent future abdominal discomfort to the patient.

Management of cardiac arrest

There has been considerable attention given in nursing texts and other teaching aids to detailed management of cardiac arrest. A brief overview will be presented with special attention to oxygen depletion and lactic acidosis. Cardiac arrest will follow a respiratory arrest when the small body stores of oxygen are depleted. The length of time involved before the heart suddenly fails to maintain a circulation in the situation depends on the patient's previous state of oxygenation, plus the state of the myocardium. The heart of the patient with high arterial blood oxygenation will be able to beat longer (up to 10 minutes) than will the heart of a patient with a low arterial oxygenation.

Cardiac arrest caused by ventricular fibrillation or ventricular asystole in the patient with cardiac disease is well known as a cause of death. Fortunately, however, early recognition of life-threatening arrhythmias by well-trained nurses, new techniques for monitoring left ventricular function, and prompt reversal of ventricular fibrillation are doing much to reduce patient mortality from this cause. Of course, cardiac arrest may occur in many other instances, particularly in patients in critical care areas. The incidence of life-threatening arrhythmias is greatly increased in patients in respiratory failure, and it now appears that any patient undergoing intensive care should have the benefit of constant cardiac monitoring equipment.

Treatment. Respiratory arrest follows cardiac arrest within seconds, and cardiac and respiratory resuscitation must be started immediately and simultaneously to save the patient's life. The patient becomes cyanotic, two or more pulses are absent (femoral and carotid), and the pupils become dilated and lose their reaction to light. The three main objectives in resuscitative measures are to:
1. Deliver oxygenated blood to the tissues
2. Restore effective cardiac contractions
3. Correct acidosis

A brief outline of procedures for management of the cardiac arrest is presented in the following list.

BRIEF OUTLINE FOR MANAGEMENT OF CARDIAC ARREST

1. Call for help and start timing.
2. Establish an airway; at the same time palpate the carotid pulse.
3. If the pulse is absent, give a sharp blow to the precordium to restore heart action.
4. If the patient is not breathing, give four quick lung inflations and establish basic CPR (five chest compressions followed by two quick lung inflations). Mouth-to-mouth ventilation or ventilating bag with mask may be used.
5. When help arrives, two-person CPR is established; one person delivers *five* chest compressions to the second person's *one* lung inflation.
6. Limb leads are attached to the patient, and cardiac monitoring is started. Observe the rhythm.
7. The defibrillator is set up.
8. An intravenous infusion is set up (if not running).
9. Drugs are prepared for administration.
10. Arterial blood is drawn for analysis as soon as possible.

Physiologic considerations. Cardiac arrest is associated with decreased delivery of oxygen and nutrients to the tissues and causes cellular hypoxia and anaerobic metabolism. This results in metabolic acidosis because of the formation and accumulation of lactic acid, since it cannot be directly blown off by the lungs. Plasma bicarbonate rapidly falls as the body attempts to correct the acidosis and restore the rapidly falling arterial pH. A respiratory acidosis may become superimposed on the metabolic acidosis if ventilation is not restored. Acidosis depresses myocardial contractility, causes potassium to leak out of the cells, and causes many other changes in cellular function.

Oxygen is required for aerobic metabolism, which produces the high-energy phosphate bonds essential to cellular function (Chapter 1). In cardiac arrest, tissue hypoxia is severe because of reduction in systemic capillary blood flow, inadequate tissue perfusion, and reduction in oxygen being transported. In response to oxygen lack the cells revert to the much less efficient emergency pathway that requires no oxygen—anaerobic metabolism of glucose (glycolysis), the end product of which is lactic acid. The result of this emergency process is little energy for cellular work (only 2 molecules of ATP from 1 molecule of glucose instead of 38 molecules as in aerobic metabolism) and the liberation of large amounts of the very strong lactic acid. Severe metabolic acidosis therefore results.

The effects of hypoxia and acidemia on cellular function are important. Normal oxidative processes cannot proceed, and the potassium electrolyte pump, which requires energy to work, fails. Therefore potassium, an important cation, leaks out, raising the serum levels of potassium and thus increasing the danger of arrhythmias. Acidemia and hyperkalemia both impair myocardial contractility, and favor ventricular fibrillation. A vicious cycle of events is thereby set up, which by its nature interferes with resuscitative efforts. A respiratory acidosis, which soon becomes superimposed on the metabolic acidosis, further adds to the problem.

To break the cycle, oxygenation and circulation must be restored. The lactic acid must be neutralized with large amounts of sodium bicarbonate, and the respiratory acid (CO_2) must be removed by effective ventilation.

CHRONIC OBSTRUCTIVE PULMONARY DISEASE

Patients with chronic obstructive pulmonary disease (COPD) include patients with chronic bronchitis, pulmonary emphysema, and bronchial asthma (Chapter 6). Such patients are usually admitted to the respiratory intensive care unit following an acute exacerbation of their disease, which is generally predisposed by one of the following events: a respiratory infection, sedation, uncontrolled oxygen therapy, reaction to heavy atmospheric pollution, or in the case of the asthmatic patient an attack unresponsive to normal treatment, which progresses to status asthmaticus.

Chronic bronchitis and pulmonary emphysema

Airways obstruction is a major characteristic of chronic obstructive pulmonary disease and may become markedly increased because of increases in pulmonary secretions. The result is that the patient has to increase his work of breathing to overcome the additional airways resistance. Abnormalities of ventilation–blood flow relationships increase as does the amount of wasted ventilation. Patients with chronic bronchitis or pulmonary emphysema or a combination of both are generally in a delicate respiratory balance, which may be tilted easily toward respiratory failure. It is not unusual to find such a patient admitted to the respiratory intensive care unit with a bout of pneumonia that he acquired during hospitalization for some other ailment. This illustrates the absolute necessity for care geared to prevention of respiratory complications.

Signs and symptoms. On admission the patient is usually distressed and dyspneic with obvious signs of increased work of breathing, such as extensive use of accessory muscles of respiration and prolongation of the expiratory phase of respiration characterized by pursed-lip breathing. Signs and symptoms of hypoxia and hypercapnia may be present. Distention of neck veins and pitting edema may be observed in the patient with cor pulmonale. The patient frequently limits his fluid intake because of persistent coughing; the resultant dehydration causes thickening of secretions, which may be copious in the presence of infection.

Diagnostic procedures. *Arterial blood gas analysis* is essential to assessment of (1) the degree of hypoxemia, (2) the degree of hypercapnia, and (3) the severity of the acid-base disturbance. Many patients with chronic obstructive pulmonary disease are "sixty-sixty" people. They have an arterial Po_2 of 60 mm Hg (normal is 90 to 100) and an arterial Pco_2 of 60 mm Hg (normal is 40). An acute exacerbation of the disease results in a further increase in carbon dioxide and a concomitant fall in arterial Po_2. In this situation the degree of hypoxia may be severe enough to result in a metabolic acidosis caused by the accumulation of lactic acid resulting from anaerobic metabolism. Renal compensation for chronic elevation of carbon dioxide (respiratory acidosis) results in an elevated bicarbonate level, which brings the pH within normal limits. In this situation the superimposed metabolic acidosis on the chronic respiratory acidosis will be reflected as a decrease in pH and bicarbonate and an elevated carbon dioxide level.

Simple *tests of pulmonary function* can be measured at the bedside. Vital capacity and forced expiratory volume will provide information on the degree of airways obstruction and loss of vital capacity. This reflects the reserve the patient has to work with.

A *chest x-ray examination* will reveal the presence of the destructive changes of emphysema, pleural effusion, atelectasis, or pneumothorax. Information on the size and position of the heart and great vessels plus the position of the diaphragm is also provided.

Laboratory examinations include sputum smear, measurement of hemoglobin and hematocrit, white cell count, serum electrolytes, and blood urea. Urinalysis is usually routine. In patients with chronic obstructive pulmonary disease, hemoglobin and hematocrit levels are often elevated because of secondary polycythemia resulting from chronic hypoxia. White cell count will be elevated in the presence of infection; changes in electrolytes, particularly potassium and sodium, occur frequently because of acid-base irregularities or the use of diuretics.

Electrocardiographic changes may suggest evidence of previous chronic respiratory failure and cor pulmonale.

A complete history and physical examination of the patient are carried out, noting particularly general physical and mental status of the patient, quality of breath sounds, and changes in anatomic integrity of the thorax.

Treatment. The principles of treatment employed in managing a patient suffering an acute exacerbation of chronic obstructive pulmonary disease are (1) relief of hypoxia, (2) restoration of adequate alveolar ventilation, and (3) treatment of infection.

Relief of hypoxia is accomplished in less severe respiratory failure from chronic obstructive pulmonary disease by controlled oxygen therapy (Chapter 8). Low-flow oxygen therapy of 1 to 2 liters should be administered initially, until blood gas determinations reveal the degree of hypoxemia and hypercapnia present. It is absolutely vital that these patients are nursed where constant supervision is available. Some well-meaning person may think that the oxygen delivery system is not working correctly because the flow rate is so low and will increase it. This may kill the patient. Signs should be well posted to prevent this mishap, and all who have patient contact should be made aware of this danger.

Because the patient with chronic obstructive pulmonary disease frequently has a hypoxic drive to respiration, a further elevation of arterial PCO_2 will usually follow the administration of oxygen. This rise will generally occur over the first 2 hours after initiation of therapy and may be in a range of 10 to 30 mm Hg. If the patient has a marked elevation of arterial PCO_2 to begin with (80 mm Hg), this further increase may produce carbon dioxide narcosis. The patient should be carefully observed for changes in mental status, such as progressive drowsiness. Frequent monitoring of arterial blood gases is carried out prior to and for the first 24 hours following controlled oxygen therapy in these patients.

Restoration of adequate alveolar ventilation is essential to the relief of hypercapnia, and therapy aimed toward this goal should be initiated immediately. This is accomplished through vigorous chest physiotherapy to remove secretions, the use of bronchodilators to relieve bronchospasm, IPPB therapy to aerate the alveoli, systemic and local humidification to dilute pulmonary secretions, and the use of mucolytic agents to reduce sputum viscosity. The majority of patients in respiratory failure from chronic obstructive pulmonary disease do not require intubation and assisted ventilation if the aforementioned therapies are vigorously instituted. This does not mean, however, that they should be nursed in anything less than a respiratory intensive care setting. Such therapy demands the attendance of a skilled respiratory care team on a 24-hour basis.

IPPB therapy is administered frequently to the patient with an acute exacerbation of his disease to remove carbon dioxide and to fully aerate alveoli. Indeed, half-hourly or hourly treatments for 15 minutes are often required to achieve this. Since the patient with chronic obstructive pulmonary disease frequently has air trapping because of bronchiolar collapse during the expiratory phase of respiration, the use of a *retard cap* placed over the exhalation opening of the IPPB machine is required. This provides a back pressure during expiration, which prevents airways collapse and allows the patient a more complete exhalation.

Because of the neurologic changes resulting from hypoxemia and hypercapnia, the patient with chronic obstructive pulmonary disease is not always easy to nurse. A sympathetic, understanding approach and a firm desire to maintain adequate therapy are essential to get the patient over the acute phase of respiratory failure. The patient may be drowsy yet must be aroused frequently to cough and remove secretions. Hypoventilation is exacerbated by sleep, which at this stage is dangerous to the patient. When a patient becomes confused, angry, or noisy, it is better to check his arterial blood gases and to give him an IPPB treatment if possible. Usually the blood gases will reveal a marked increase in Pco_2 and decrease in Po_2, which is why the patient's behavior is strange. Tranquilizers or sedation of any kind should not be given to these patients to quiet them.

When the arterial Pco_2 continues to rise despite vigorous therapy, endotracheal intubation and mechanical ventilation are generally instituted. Skilled management is required because the patient usually has both reduced lung and thoracic compliance because of anatomic changes in the thorax and elastic changes in lung tissue. There is also increased airways resistance caused by obstruction and spasm. Changes in cardiac function are frequently present, and there are marked increases in physiologic dead space. Several IPPB machines deliver high concentrations of oxygen when they are set at "air dilution." Compressed air or strictly controlled oxygen delivery is required in management of these patients because of their hypoxic drive to respiration. Patients with chronic obstructive pulmonary disease are used to an arterial Po_2 of 60 mm Hg or slightly above, and if a Pa_{O_2} of 70 to 80 mm Hg is maintained with mechanical ventilation, this is considered adequate. Such a level provides a margin of safety during suctioning or in the event of cardiac arrest.

Prognosis. Chronic obstructive pulmonary disease cannot be cured, but with sufficient physical and psychosocial rehabilitation these patients can be made to feel they are useful members of society and less of a burden to their families. The aid of all health team members is needed—dieticians to see that the patient's meals are what he enjoys and to supply small frequent meals, physiotherapists to train the patient in special breathing techniques, respiratory therapists to provide instruction in home IPPB machines and the use of bronchodilators, plus social workers and psychiatrists as needed. Nurses at the bedside can contribute in all areas. Because of their constant care of the patient, they are the prime movers in the physical and psychosocial rehabilitation that is so essential to these patients.

Status asthmaticus

Severe respiratory distress may occur in the patient with bronchial asthma when the attack is prolonged and unresponsive to the usual therapies. Status asthmaticus is a medical emergency from which over 2,000 patients a year die. It has been said of status asthmaticus, "The longer it lasts the worse it gets, the worse it gets the longer it lasts." In my own experience with patients with asthma, this statement certainly holds true.

The precipitating event to status asthmaticus may be a respiratory infection, exposure to a specific allergen, extreme changes in temperature (hot or cold), or heavy atmospheric pollution. Not infrequently the attack may be predisposed by a see-saw approach to therapy. For example, on the days the patient feels well, he may not take his medication, and then when he has a "bad day," he may take more than is required in an attempt to stop the wheezing and discomfort.

Signs and symptoms. The patient in status asthmaticus is usually pale, dyspneic, distressed, and fighting for every breath. A marked increase in the work of breathing is observed. Severe wheezing, which is audible across the room, may be present, or the chest may be "silent" because of severe airway narrowing and blockage with mucus plugs. The patient uses the accessory muscles of respiration, and the expiratory phase of respiration is prolonged. Tachycardia is frequently present because of excessive use of bronchodilator aerosols and the severe apprehension the condition evokes. Signs of dehydration, exhaustion, and cyanosis may also be observed.

Diagnostic procedures. Arterial blood gas analysis is required to determine the degree of hypoxemia and the acid-base status of the patient. The patient usually has a degree of hypoxemia because of regional hypoventilation relative to perfusion that is caused by accumulated secretions and airways obstruction. Metabolic changes result in these patients having acidemia with a reduction in pH. A sudden rise in P_{CO_2} often occurs as the patient's condition progresses to respiratory failure, and this compounds the acidosis.

Simple tests of pulmonary function reveal a marked reduction in vital capacity, severe reduction of forced expiratory volume, and maximal expiratory flow rate due to profound bronchial spasm, mucus plugs, and inflammation and edema of the airway walls.

Chest x-ray examination will reveal any changes caused by atelectasis, pneumonia, or pneumothorax (such complications may be present).

Laboratory studies will include routine electrolyte determination, urinalysis, sputum smear, hemoglobin and hematocrit determination, and a white blood cell count (WBC). Eosinophils, which normally make up from 1% to 4% of the white count, are increased dramatically during an attack of asthma.

Treatment. Immediate treatment is required to relieve bronchial muscle spasm, clear secretions, correct acidosis, correct hypoxemia, and alleviate the patient's apprehension and fear.

Intravenous aminophylline is administered *slowly* as an initial dose of 500 mg or 5 to 6 mg/kg of body weight. The patient usually experiences some relief immediately from this therapy. An intravenous infusion is generally set up for fluid replacement and continuous aminophylline infusion. The dose is usually 0.9 mg/kg each hour for a 24-hour period. Heavy doses of *steroids* are required. For example, from 60 to 80 mg of prednisolone are given daily following an initial intravenous injection of methylprednisolone. Their action is to reduce inflammation and block the allergic reaction at the mast cell site.

Measurement of serum theophylline concentrations has proved to be of value in monitoring the dosage of theophylline and its derivatives for patients. Many clinical laboratories now have the equipment available for such analysis.

Oxygen therapy with high humidification is required to relieve hypoxemia and to liquefy secretions. Low-flow controlled therapy should be given until it is determined that there is no chronic hypercapnia and hypoxemia. Higher concentrations (50% to 70%) may be given otherwise. Vigorous chest physiotherapy is required to remove secretions, and an antibiotic is required for an infection.

Acidosis is corrected by restoring ventilation to remove carbon dioxide (respiratory component) and by administering sodium bicarbonate to correct the metabolic component. Correction of acidosis in the asthmatic patient, it appears, has the advantage of improving the response of bronchial muscle to bronchodilators because increased hydrogen ion concentrations have been found to reduce the sensitivity of the bronchial muscle to bronchodilators.

Apprehension and anxiety are frequent symptoms experienced by the asthmatic patient during a severe attack. This not only results from the feelings wrought by the condition but from the side effects of the drugs used. Sedation and tranquilizers are often required to relieve these symptoms, but the dosage is usually small and well controlled because of the depressant effect on respiration. Nurses should constantly reassure the patient and carefully control the patient's environment. The patient should be protected from allergic or other stimuli that may precipitate a further attack. In some instances this may lead to restricting the visiting rights of certain family members.

Mechanical ventilation with endotracheal intubation is required to treat the patient with status asthmaticus when all conventional therapy fails. Inflation pressures as high as 80 to 100 cm of water are required to overcome the marked increase in airways resistance. Another problem that may arise with the asthmatic patient is a difficulty in synchronizing the ventilator with the patient because there is usually no interference with the normal drive to respiration. A combination of high inflation pressures, increased intrathoracic pressure, and increased intra-alveolar pressure (due to increased airways resistance during expiration) cause impairment in venous return to the heart, a fall in cardiac output, and hypotension.

Prognosis. A severe attack of asthma is usually broken during the first 24 to 48 hours of therapy, and the patient will be able to be transferred from the respiratory intensive care unit. The time spent on the unit will be longer if the patient requires intubation and mechanical ventilation. Protecting the patient from exposure to the offending stimuli may reduce the frequency of the attacks. Careful instruction of the patient in the use of bronchodilators is important. Their overuse renders them ineffective in bringing relief; it is most important, however, to maintain adequate blood levels with *regular* administration.

COR PULMONALE

Heart failure secondary to pulmonary disease is known as cor pulmonale. This may result from primary abnormalities of (1) the lungs, (2) the pulmonary vasculature, or (3) pulmonary gas exchange. Although cor pulmonale most commonly develops in patients with chronic lung diseases, it may also develop in a number of disorders that do not affect the lung directly but produce abnormalities in gas exchange and ventilatory mechanics. For example, cor pulmonale may develop with neuromuscular disorders that affect respiratory muscle function or with extreme obesity (Chapter 6). The primary mechanisms of cor pulmonale are pulmonary hypertension and hypoxemia with or without hypercapnia.

The pulmonary circulation is a low-pressure and low-resistance system (Chapter 4). The pressure in the right ventricle and pulmonary capillaries is far less than in the left ventricle and capillaries of the systemic circulation. The abnormalities of structure and function of the heart in cor pulmonale are caused by an increase in the work of the right ventricle, which results from an increase in pulmonary vascular resistance. The right ventricle must work harder to pump the normal cardiac output through the pulmonary circulation. An increase in pulmonary vascular resistance may be brought about by one or all of the following: (1) anatomic reduction of the pulmonary vascular bed, (2) pulmonary vasoconstriction, or (3) abnormalities of ventilatory mechanics.

Patients with chronic obstructive pulmonary disease, particularly pulmonary emphysema, frequently have all the predisposing factors to pulmonary vascular resistance. Pulmonary emphysematous destructive changes result in a loss of pulmonary capillaries. Alveolar hypoxia and respiratory acidosis cause pulmonary vasoconstriction, and abnormalities of ventilatory mechanics associated with obstructive disease bring about compression of the pulmonary capillaries because of increases in alveolar pressure. An increase in the viscosity of the blood, due to the secondary polycythemia of chronic obstructive pulmonary disease, may also contribute to pulmonary hypertension and its associated right ventricular strain.

Signs and symptoms. Although there are many other conditions that result in cor pulmonale, from 70% to 75% of cases in the United States occur in patients with chronic obstructive pulmonary disease. On admission these patients will usually give a 5- to 10-year history of such disease; hence the clinical manifestations frequently overlap. The major factors of right heart failure are congestive changes, which manifest themselves as distended neck veins and peripheral edema. The patient's chief complaint is usually dyspnea, particularly on exertion, and cough.

Diagnostic procedures. The tests for cor pulmonale are the same as for chronic obstructive pulmonary disease. Particular attention is paid to the history, physical examination, chest x ray, and electrocardiogram.

Chest x-ray examination will reveal anatomic enlargement of the heart and engorgement of the pulmonary artery. Pleural effusion because of extravasation of fluid into the pleural cavity (a result of venous congestion) may also be seen.

The *electrocardiograph* demonstrates altered spatial orientation of the heart and changes resulting from right ventricular and right atrial hypertrophy.

Physical examination for congestive changes is most important. Pitting edema is usually observed and, in the presence of tricuspid insufficiency, hepatomegaly or ascites may be seen. The patient may have a history of either pulmonary or cardiac disease.

Treatment. Improvement in alveolar ventilation, relief of hypoxemia, and treatment of edema are major considerations in treatment of the patient with cor pulmonale. The course of treatment, of course, will vary depending on the underlying disorder. Bronchial toilet for removal of secretions (chest physiotherapy, IPPB, and humidification) and bronchodilators for the relief of bronchospasm are therapies to improve alveolar ventilation. In turn, the improved ventilation will lessen vasoconstriction by relieving respiratory acidosis and reducing alveolar pressure. Relief of hypoxemia with controlled oxygen therapy will also reduce vasoconstriction. The result is a reduction in pulmonary hypertension and right ventricular strain. Digitalis is used to increase (1) the force of cardiac contraction, (2) the time of ventricular filling, and (3) the stroke volume of the heart. All of these factors are important in treating heart failure.

Edema is controlled by restricting fluid and sodium intake and by the use of diuretics. These diuretics include the thiazides (Diuril or Hydrodiuril); furosemide (Lasix); ethacrynic acid (Edecrin); or aldosterone antagonists, such as spironolactone (Aldactone) and triamterene (Dyrenium).

Serial determinations of fluid electrolytes are important in patients receiving diuretics because of the changes they bring about in urinary electrolyte excretion, particularly of sodium, potassium, chloride, and bicarbonate. Digitalis toxicity may result in the presence of potassium deficiency (hypokalemia). This may be prevented by the administration of potassium chloride when the thiazides or furosemide is used. The electrolyte effects of diuretics should also be remembered when the acid-base status of the patient is examined.

Phlebotomy is used to reduce blood volume in patients with severe polycythemia (hematocrit level greater than 60%). This treatment is usually performed over a few days by removing from 200 to 300 ml of blood each day, which gradually reduces the red cell mass. The concomitant reduction in blood viscosity has the advantage of reducing the work of the right ventricle. Carbonic anhydrase inhibitors have been used in certain cases because of their diuretic effect and their reduction of carbon dioxide through inhibition of carbon dioxide transport and increased renal excretion of bicarbonate.

Daily weights and maintenance of strict fluid balance are essential elements of nursing care, as are frequent examination of the patient for signs of increased edema and cardiac monitoring for early recognition of arrhythmias associated with the underlying cardiac mechanism or drug administration. General physical and psychosocial elements of nursing care are also administered.

Prognosis. There appear to be few statistics on the survival rate of patients with cor pulmonale. Apparently patients who progress to congestive heart failure have a limited life expectancy, whereas patients having a milder form of cardiac involvement may survive for many years. Studies reveal that improved therapeutic measures have helped patients over the crisis of respiratory failure associated with infections or a period of heart failure, doing much to extend life expectancy.

ACUTE PULMONARY EDEMA

Acute pulmonary edema in its full stage is a life-threatening clinical emergency. It may result from left ventricular failure, cor pulmonale, local irritation of the alveoli (irritant gases or burns), or shock conditions associated with the adult respiratory distress syndrome or hypervolemia. The mechanisms of pulmonary edema are complex and still not clearly understood. It appears that pulmonary edema is of three types: intracellular, interstitial, and intra-alveolar. The intra-alveolar type is known as acute pulmonary edema.

Transudation of fluid into the alveoli may occur with critical elevations of the pulmonary capillary pressure (Chapter 4) but also depends on the permeability of the alveolar capillary membrane and other factors. For example, the fatty acids resulting from fat emboli are known to result in severe pulmonary edema, as are certain neurogenic factors.

The pressure in the pulmonary capillaries is estimated at 6 mm Hg. When transudation of fluid occurs into the alveoli, a "critical" elevation of pulmonary capillary pressure, which exceeds the colloid osmotic pressure of 25 mm Hg, is frequently present. This results in fluid being forced into the alveoli, causing acute pulmonary edema (intra-alveolar). One cause of the increased pulmonary capillary pressure is the dam effect from the left ventricle back through the pulmonary circulation present in left ventricular failure and valvular disease. (See Chapter 4.)

Signs and symptoms. A feeling of anxiety by the patient may be the only warning sign of acute pulmonary edema, which is rapidly followed by dyspnea, orthopnea, wheezing, pallor, and bubbling rales. Copious amounts of blood-stained frothy sputum are expectorated. Foaming of sputum and bubbling rales are produced as the patient increases his respiratory rate in an attempt to get more air. This rapid mixture of air with the alveolar fluid produces the froth. Movement of fluid in the airways causes bubbling rales, which are audible without a stethoscope as noisy, moist, crackling respirations. As the condition worsens, severe hypoxia causes the patient to become cyanotic and confused. If therapy is not instituted immediately, death may rapidly approach.

Treatment. Acute pulmonary edema is a ghastly experience for the patient and results in extreme mental anxiety. This is usually relieved with the administration of *morphine sulfate*, 8 to 15 mg, given intravenously (initially). Morphine sulfate sedates the patient, provides muscle relaxation and, most importantly, inhibits mechanisms that contribute to pulonary edema. However, because morphine sulfate is a respiratory depressant, the drug must be administered with extreme caution to patients with underlying respiratory disease.

Aminophylline, 250 to 500 mg, administered by slow intravenous injection is effective in reducing bronchospasm and improving cardiovascular function. It improves cardiac output and lowers venous pressure by reducing muscle spasm of the blood vessels.

Immediate measures to *relieve hypoxia and retard venous return* (to reduce pressures in the pulmonary capillaries) are instituted by special intermittent positive pressure breathing techniques. High oxygen concentrations are administered initially, because of the extreme widening of the diffusion pathway. IPPB therapy is used in this situation to generate high intrathoracic pressures by using high inflation pressures or rates of flow. This maintains high pressures at end inspiration to block venous return. The result is improved ventilation and oxygenation and a decrease in the edema. Rotating tourniquets or phlebotomy are also measures used to retard venous return.

Treatment of the underlying mechanism of acute pulmonary edema has important bearing on special therapeutic factors (for example, the use of digitalis in the presence of cardiac failure). Because acute pulmonary edema can occur in a variety of conditions, the therapeutic measures just described are those employed generally in most situations.

ADULT RESPIRATORY DISTRESS SYNDROME

Attention has been directed to a group of conditions that result in pathophysiologic changes in *normal* adult lungs, which bear remarkable similarity to those found in the respiratory distress syndrome of the newborn. "Shock lung," "postperfusion lung," and several other names were initially given to the disorders, but the *adult respiratory distress syndrome* (ARDS) is now generally accepted terminology.

Etiology. A list of causes of the adult respiratory distress syndrome were presented in Table 10, p. 141. It is a major cause of hypoxemic respiratory failure. These patients' lungs are normal initially. The pathophysiologic changes that occur arise from either (1) massive trauma elsewhere in the body, such as severe burns, crush injuries (which may include pulmonary contusion), or injury sustained in combat or (2) changes arising from oxygen toxicity, fat embolism, rapid excessive transfusion, diffuse capillary leak syndrome, viral pneumonia, cerebral hypoxia, or any other condition that results in severe shock.

Signs and symptoms. In many instances the onset of the syndrome occurs 48 to 72 hours following initial treatment of the underlying condition. It is heralded by dyspnea, tachypnea, reduction in vital capacity due to reduction in compliance, and impairment of gas exchange (which at first is a moderate reduction in arterial PO_2). As the condition continues, the physiologic changes become more serious, and the arterial PO_2 continues to decrease despite all efforts to administer and maintain a satisfactory inspired-oxygen concentration. Radiologic changes are seen as patchy infiltrates, which progress to opacity of the lung; the chest film resembles a snowstorm.

When nursing a patient in respiratory failure who may be developing the adult respiratory distress syndrome, the two earliest signs that the nurse may observe are tachypnea and the presence of basilar rales heard late in inspiration.

Pathogenesis. Changes in the lung at the alveolar capillary level are great; these include interstitial edema, intra-alveolar pulmonary edema, intra-alveolar hemorrhages, and hyaline membrane. The pulmonary capillaries become congested and their permeability increases. There is a severe ventilation-perfusion abnormality. Carbon dioxide retention does not occur until the end stages of the disease process because it is more soluble and therefore can traverse the diffusion pathway. A decrease in pulmonary surfactant caused by hypoxia and the general "wetness" of the alveoli results in the need for more pressure to open them.

Treatment. Main treatment concepts are based on maintaining an adequate Po_2 (>50 mm Hg). This is not always easy to do without giving high concentrations of oxygen, which may damage an already injured lung. Inspired oxygen concentrations of 0.70 (FI_{O_2}) or less are used wherever possible. Mechanical support to respiration is frequently required to deliver the high inflation pressures needed to overcome the marked decrease in compliance. To provide better distribution of ventilation, the application of positive end-expiratory pressure (PEEP) or continuous positive airway pressure (CPAP) is frequently used.

The use of PEEP has proved to be of value because it reduces the wide alveolar-arterial oxygen tension differences that occur in patients with the adult respiratory distress syndrome and thus permits a reduction in FI_{O_2}.

It appears that the degree of increase in arterial oxygen tension when positive end-expiratory pressure is applied is related to the resultant increases in lung volume. For example, researchers have shown that an increase in functional residual capacity of 1.18 liters was brought about by applying a PEEP of 13 cm of water. The result was an increase in arterial Po_2 of 179 mm Hg, whereas a PEEP of 5 cm of water resulted in an increase in FRC of 0.35 liters and an increase in arterial Po_2 of 63 mm Hg. These patients were receiving 70% oxygen—a partial pressure of inspired oxygen of 499 mm Hg (70% of 760 − 47) (Chapter 5).

An effort is made to keep the lung dry by fluid restriction and the use of diuretics. This type of therapy is carefully controlled so that the intravascular volume is not suddenly reduced, causing further cardiopulmonary complications. This and other therapies such as the use of colloids (albumin and dextran 40 or dextran 70) are directed at pulling the fluid from the pulmonary interstitial space.

The patient with adult respiratory distress syndrome requires skilled nursing care, using many of the monitoring techniques described in Chapter 11 and the therapies described in other chapters to prevent further complications.

Successful use has been made in treatment of ARDS of a membrane oxygenator to provide extracorporeal oxygenation until the lungs themselves can provide adequate gas exchange. In an attempt to save patients' lives, patients have been transferred to facilities where such services are available. There are medical teams that have taken themselves and their equipment to the patients' hospital bedside.

Prognosis. The mortality rate from adult respiratory distress syndrome at present is high. These are life-threatening disorders that occur rapidly, and the mechanisms are not entirely understood. Reports on patients who have survived the syndrome show that there is a significant reduction in vital capacity, reduction in compliance, and a diffusion defect that persists for several months following illness. Gradual restoration of pulmonary function takes place as the months pass, but as far as is known the patient's lungs do not return to normal. Research into the syndrome mechanisms continues.

CHEST INJURIES

Patients with multiple chest injuries are being seen in intensive care units in ever-increasing numbers. Such injuries are usually sustained in major traffic or industrial accidents or in attempted suicide or homicide. Chest trauma is particularly hazardous because of the number of vital structures contained within the thoracic cavity.

Anatomic and physiologic considerations

Because of the complexity of intrathoracic and extrathoracic function, the anatomic location of the injury will influence to a degree the physiologic process. Injuries to the chest can vary from a mild injury involving simple rib fracture to the most severe mechanical instability of the chest wall, flail chest.

Flail chest. Mechanical instability of the chest wall results from either multiple rib fractures or fractures of the ribs and sternum, often with separation at the costochondral junctions. These cause large areas of the chest wall to be free floating, which in turn results in *paradoxical respiration.* The unstable chest is sucked in during inspiration instead of being pulled out, and the underlying lung is unable to inflate. Marked impairment in ventilation occurs, reflected by hypoxia, hypercapnia, and an increased work of breathing.

Lung contusion. Crushing and bruising of the lung is known as contusion. It can be caused by a severe blow to the chest without rib or sternal fracture. Because of damage to the alveolar structures, lung contusion leads to atelectasis and airways obstruction from plugging of bronchioles by blood and edema fluid. Ventilation is impaired because of the reduction in lung compliance.

Lung compression. Pneumothorax, hemothorax, or pleural effusion cause compression of the lung, which further impairs respiratory function and leads to atelectatic changes in the lung by limiting alveolar expansion.

Tension pneumothorax. Tension pneumothorax occurs in the presence of sucking wounds of the chest or by way of a communication resulting from a damaged trachea or bronchus. Air enters the pleural space on inspiration but cannot escape on expiration because of a one-way valve mechanism set up by a tissue flap that seals the wound during expiration. This leads to a build-up of air in the intrapleural space, which compresses the lung, usually shifting it toward the mediastinum. Displacement of mediastinal structures may follow. Tension pneumothorax not infrequently develops in patients with chest injuries during the first few hours of mechanical ventilation as air is forced into the pleural space through unknown damaged areas.

Cardiac injury. Crush injuries of the chest may also result in contusion of the heart and great vessels. Complications such as loss of myocardial integrity or cardiac tamponade can arise.

Rupture of major structures. Rupture of vital structures such as the trachea, a bronchus, the thoracic aorta, or the diaphragm may occur. Damage to the trachea or bronchi may lead to complications such as tension pneumothorax, bronchopleural fistula, or subcutaneous emphysema. Abdominal contents may herniate through a torn diaphragm.

The patient with chest injuries not infrequently suffers severe pain, which further reduces effective alveolar ventilation. Reduction in blood volume from hemorrhage, accompanied by hypotension compounded by hypoxia will lead to cardiorespiratory failure.

Treatment

Treatment objectives are to establish effective alveolar ventilation, to relieve hypoxia, and to maintain cardiac output and blood pressure. Surgical repair of the trachea or other major structures is then generally undertaken. *Mild chest injuries* with simple rib fracture and no flail chest can usually be treated with analgesics or intercostal nerve blocks for the relief of pain, oxygen therapy, and chest physiotherapy. Deep breathing and coughing are essential to prevent respiratory complications in these patients. Because of fear and pain, patients with even mild injuries will limit their respiratory movements. When the injury to the chest is mild but the patient has interference with normal respiratory function because of either cerebral trauma or preexisting lung disease, ventilator support by way of an endotracheal tube may be indicated to clear secretions. A chest x-ray is obtained in all patients to pinpoint the location and degree of injury.

Severe chest injuries with marked flail chest are treated promptly. The airway is cleared, an endotracheal tube is passed, and ventilation is controlled with positive-pressure controlled ventilation. The patient is not permitted to self-cycle the ventilator because of paradoxical chest movement. An intravenous infusion is started, and a central venous catheter is passed into the vena cava to monitor fluid load. Hemorrhage in patients with chest injuries requires that a sample of blood be typed and cross-matched for blood transfusions. Arterial blood gases are usually analyzed to ascertain ventilatory status.

Treatment of pneumothorax when present is immediate; a chest tube is inserted into the second intercostal space anteriorly with a trocar and affixed to the skin. A running suture is used to allow the skin to be drawn around the tube to prevent leakage of air through the incision. A Vaseline gauze dressing is used to make an additional seal. The chest tube is then attached to an underwater-seal drainage system. Drainage of blood or other fluid from the chest will require insertion of a second chest tube in a more dependent area.

The prevalence of recurrent pneumothorax, tension pneumothorax, or hemothorax in patients with chest injuries requires that a thoracentesis tray, equipped with a large enough thoracotomy trocar to permit passage of a chest tube, be at the bedside of the patient with chest injuries at all times.

Patients with chest injuries require intensive nursing care and mechanical ventilation over prolonged periods of time. Several chest tubes may be in situ, which demand constant attention to the size of air leaks and the quantity and nature of chest drainage. All the bedside monitoring techniques described previously apply to the care of the patient with chest injuries, plus more frequent examination and auscultation of the chest for changes in thoracic movement and breath sounds. Diminished breath sounds and fixation of the chest on one side may be the first signs of tension pneumothorax in the patient undergoing controlled mechanical ventilation. Pain is relieved with frequent small doses of a sedative in order to avoid respiratory depression. Intercostal nerve blocks with local anesthesia also bring about substantial relief from pain.

Severe multiple trauma brings with it all the hazards of immobility: (1) respiratory complications such as atelectasis, infection, or edema and (2) embolization from fat, debris, or clotted elements. The patient's position should be frequently changed whenever possible, range-of-motion exercises conducted, and periodic hyperinflation of the lung carried out to prevent complications.

REFERENCES

Gracy, D. R.: Adult respiratory distress syndrome, Heart Lung 4:280-284, 1975.

Hill, J. D., et al.: Prolonged extracorporeal oxygenation, for acute posttraumatic respiratory failure: shock lung syndrome, N. Engl. J. Med. **286:**629-634, 1972.

Hudson, L. D.: The acute management of the chronic airway obstruction patient, Heart Lung 3(1):93-96, 1974.

Petty, T. L.: Acute airways obstruction and status asthmaticus (abstract), 14th Annual Symposium on Critical Care Medicine, San Francisco, 1976.

Petty, T. L., and Ashbaugh, D. G.: The adult respiratory distress syndrome, Chest **60:**233-239, 1971.

Reed, C. E., and Siegel, S. E., editors: Asthma: medicom learning system, Palo Alto, 1974, Syntex Laboratories.

Robin, E. D., and Guadio, R.: Cor pulmonale, Disease-a-month, May, 1970.

Robin, E. D., Cross, C. E., and Zelis, R.: Pulmonary edema, N. Engl. J. Med. **288:**239-246, 1973.

Rogers, R. M., Weiler, C., and Ruppenthal, B.: The impact of the respiratory intensive care unit on survival of patients with acute respiratory failure, Heart Lung 1(4):475-480, 1972.

Secor, J.: Patient care in respiratory problems: monograph in clinical nursing-1, Philadelphia, 1969, W. B. Saunders Co.

Shoemaker, W. C.: A logarithm for resuscitation: a systematic plan for immediate care of the injured or postoperative patient, Crit. Care Med. 3:127-130, 1975.

Standards of cardiopulmonary resuscitation (CPR) emergency cardiac care (ECC) J.A.M.A. **227:**832-869S, 1974.

Suter, P. M., Fairley, H. B., and Isenberg, M. D.: Optimum end-expiratory airway pressure in patients with acute pulmonary failure, N. Engl. J. Med. **292:**284-289, 1975.

Votteri, B. A.: Hand-operated emergency ventilating devices, Heart Lung 1:277-282, 1972.

West, J. B.: Pulmonary gas exchange in the critically ill patient, Crit. Care Med. 2:171-181, 1974.

11 / BEDSIDE MONITORING IN RESPIRATORY INTENSIVE CARE

The purpose of bedside monitoring is to observe and evaluate the patient's condition. This provides for early recognition of deterioration in the condition, permits therapeutic intervention, and establishes a permanent record of the patient's day-to-day status. Apart from the common vital signs of temperature, pulse, respiration, and systemic blood pressure, certain special monitoring techniques of cardiopulmonary function are required when caring for the critically ill respiratory patient. Many of the measurements of cardiopulmonary function to be presented in this chapter apply to any patient requiring intensive care, not just to the respiratory patient.

MEASURING AND MONITORING VENTILATION

As with any monitoring, it is advisable to have suitable charts for nurses and therapists to record their findings and measurements taken during the care of the respiratory patient. It is also advisable to keep in mind certain principles of monitoring when a particular measurement or test is carried out. A test should be (1) *specific:* it should precisely identify a pathophysiologic event; (2) *predictive:* it should warn of complications; and (3) *relevant:* it should identify disorders or complications that frequently occur in management of the respiratory patient.

Breathing frequency (f)

One of the measurements most commonly hurried or overlooked is the respiratory rate (breathing frequency). When breathing frequency is monitored, four parameters of respiration should be noted: rate, depth, pattern, and sound. The normal respiratory rate for an adult is 15 to 20 breaths a minute, with considerable variations on the low side of the normal value. A marked increase in breathing frequency (tachypnea) may be a warning of respiratory complications such as atelectasis, bronchospasm, or pulmonary edema. When the respiratory rate of a patient is counted during mechanical ventilation, the rate of the ventilator should also be checked to make sure the patient is not breathing out of phase with the ventilator. Tachypnea may also be associated with changes in the patient's respiratory status that make him "fight" the ventilator. The latter usually indicates the need for alteration in ventilator settings. Care should be taken, however, to see that there are no other factors causing this, such as accumulated secretions, change in cuff integrity, or blockage of the endotracheal or tracheostomy tube. Tachypnea may be present with hyperventilation or hypoventilation; thus any change in breathing frequency should be recorded. Changes in respiratory pattern occur in several conditions (p. 218), for example, Kussmaul respiration occurring in diabetic ketoacidosis. Respiratory depth (tidal volume) is not easily determined by simple observation, but the excursions of the patient's chest can be observed and the uniformity and degree of expansion noted. Limited thoracic expansion may be a result of anginal pain, chest injury (such as a fractured rib), or surgical trauma.

When the respiratory rate is counted, it is also important for the nurse to listen to the respiratory sounds. Wheezing associated with asthma or the bubbling rales of pulmonary edema are frequently audible without a stethoscope.

Minute volume

Tidal volume (V_T) is usually measured during the same time interval as breathing frequency so that a minute volume of ventilation ($\dot{V}_E$) can be calculated (tidal volume × frequency = minute ventilation). When a patient is undergoing mechanical ventilation, the minute volume is frequently measured using a Wright respirometer. This small clocklike device is attached to the exhalation port of a mechanical ventilator. During each patient exhalation, the volume is reflected on the dial by a pointer, which at the end of the desired period of time, will show the accumulated volume. When the tidal volume is measured using a ventilator spirometer attachment, it is important to know when it was last checked for accuracy.

Since minute volume involves measurement of tidal volume and breathing frequency, changes in either of these respiratory parameters will alter the minute volume. However, in the presence of pulmonary disease, the tidal volume may well be reduced by half and yet the respiratory frequency doubled without changing the minute volume.

$$\text{Normal } V_T \ 500 \times f \ 15 = \dot{V}_E \ 7,500 \text{ ml}$$
$$\text{Example } V_T \ 250 \times f \ 30 = \dot{V}_E \ 7,500 \text{ ml}$$

Patients with restrictive lung disease frequently have markedly reduced tidal volumes and in an attempt to compensate, tend to breathe rapidly to provide adequate ventilation each minute.

Tidal volumes that are lower than expected may result from changes in the patient's condition, such as accumulations of fluid or secretions in the lungs (reduction in lung compliance) or increased airways resistance due to spasm. Partial failure of the ventilatory equipment because of leaks in the system at the humidifier, in the tubing, or at the exhalation valve will also bring about reduction in exhaled tidal volume or cause faulty readings.

Dead space–to–tidal volume ratio

Measurement of physiologic dead space is important to determine the total wasted (dead space) ventilation or that which is ineffective in gas exchange (Chapter 4). The physician is usually interested in the ratio of tidal volume to physiologic dead space (V_D/V_T ratio), that is, the portion of the tidal volume which is truly ventilating the patient. This can be calculated from a simplified version of the physiologic dead space equation if the patient's arterial and expired carbon dioxide levels and tidal volume are known.

$$V_D/V_T = \frac{\text{Arterial } P_{CO_2} - \text{Mixed expired } CO_2}{\text{Arterial } P_{CO_2}}$$

Normally the dead space–to–tidal volume ratio does not exceed 0.3; for example, if a patient has a tidal volume of 600 ml and a physiologic dead space of 180 ml:

$$\frac{V_D}{V_T} \frac{180}{600} = 0.3$$

As either tidal volume is reduced or the amount of wasted ventilation is increased or both, the dead space–to–tidal volume ratio increases; for example, where there are ventilation-perfusion abnormalities, one may see the following:

$$\frac{V_D}{V_T} \frac{200}{400} = 0.5$$

In pulmonary disease the V_D/V_T ratio may be as high as 0.7, where only a small percentage of the tidal volume takes part in effective gas exchange. Ventilation-perfusion abnormalities increase the V_D/V_T ratio because of the increase in wasted alveolar ventilation with respect to blood flow or the reduction of blood flow with respect to ventilation, such as in cardiac disease or pulmonary emboli.

Dead space–to–tidal volume ratios are an important consideration when ventilator settings are to be selected or altered. The nurse will recall that the relationship between alveolar ventilation and levels of arterial blood carbon dioxide is almost linear. So if ventilation is halved in a patient, levels of carbon dioxide in the arterial blood will be almost doubled. Therefore alveolar ventilation ($\dot{V}_E$), Pa_{CO_2}, and V_D/V_T ratios are all linked together. There are several nomograms now available that present in graphic form those important relationships and are most useful in selecting appropriate ventilator settings to obtain the desired Pa_{CO_2} (Fig. 11-1).

The V_D/V_T nomogram was constructed using certain physiologic principles and equations that are acceptable for clinical purposes. The instructions for use of the V_D/V_T graph are as follows:

1. Patient is placed on a ventilator with spirometer attachment, and an average minute ventilation is achieved (8 to 10 liters/min).

2. After at least 30 minutes on the ventilator at this minute ventilation, an arterial blood sample is obtained and analyzed for arterial carbon dioxide tension.

3. The minute ventilation and the corresponding Pa_{CO_2} are plotted on the graph. The V_D/V_T ratio is obtained from noting the isopleth that coincides with this point.

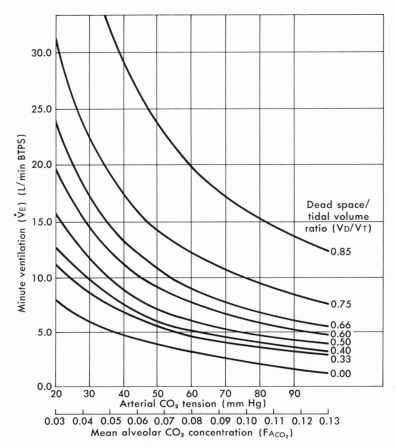

FIG. 11-1. A graphic approach to select or change minute ventilation to obtain a desired arterial P_{CO_2}, and also to estimate V_D/V_T ratios. (See text for instructions on use of the graph.) (Redrawn and printed with permission of Karlman Wasserman, M.D., Ph.D., Chief of Respiratory Physiology and Medicine, University of California, Los Angeles.)

4. To obtain the required minute ventilation to achieve any desired Pa_{CO_2}, a vertical line is drawn from the Pa_{CO_2} value on the horizontal axis to the V_D/V_T isopleth obtained in step 3. From this point a horizontal line is drawn perpendicular to the vertical axis to obtain the required minute ventilation.

5. The respirator is then adjusted by means of the pressure and rate dials to achieve the calculated minute ventilation (tidal volume × rate = minute ventilation). The rate should not exceed, if possible, 12 to 14 breaths a minute.

6. As the patient's lung problem improves, the V_D/V_T ratio will be reduced, it is hoped, requiring less minute ventilation. The ventilator should be reset to achieve this new minute ventilation by reducing either the machine pressure or rate or both. Failure to reset the ventilator could lead to overventilation and severe respiratory alkalosis with a possible fatal outcome.

7. A fall in tidal volume without a fall in machine pressure should alert the physician or nurse to the need for suctioning, bronchodilator therapy, or both.

8. The patient's course must be monitored with arterial blood gases as indicated. Whenever an arterial sample is drawn, the minute ventilation should be noted and recorded and a new V_D/V_T value obtained.

9. The new V_D/V_T ratio should be used for determining the patient's new minute ventilation.

Vital capacity

The vital capacity is defined as the volume of gas that can be expelled from the lungs by forceful effort following a maximal inspiration. Bedside measurement of vital capacity is particularly important during the postoperative period in a patient whose thorax or abdomen has been entered and also when the decision to wean a patient from mechanical ventilation is to be made. Preoperative baseline pulmonary function studies will serve as a guide for the expected vital capacity during the recovery period.

Accurate measurement of the vital capacity requires that the patient be able to follow simple instructions and that the person conducting the test is certain that the best possible results are being obtained. At least two measurements are taken, and the best value obtained is used. A Drager volumeter with a rebreathing valve can be used to measure vital capacity either by having the patient blow through a mouthpiece attached to the valve or by attaching the valve to an endotracheal tube or tracheostomy tube. A mobile spirometer or a pneumotachograph can also be used to measure the vital capacity.

The disease processes that bring about a reduction in vital capacity are presented on pp. 32-33.

Flow rates

It is useful to be able to ascertain the degree of airways obstruction by measuring the forced expiratory flow rate at the midportion of the breath FEF25-75% and also the peak flow rate. Peak flow is measured simply by use of the Wright peak flowmeter, and FEF25-75% can be measured using a spirometer or pneumotachograph. Flow-volume loops, curves, and half loops are also measured in some centers. This is accomplished by the use of a flow-sensing device (ultrasonic sensor, thermal sensor, or pneumotachograph) and some method of graphic recording, either with a pen onto calibrated paper or with computer-assisted display.

Effective dynamic compliance

A useful measurement for evaluating the work of breathing is effective dynamic compliance (EDC). This is measured by dividing the tidal volume (ml) by the peak airway pressure (cm H_2O). For example, if a patient has a tidal volume of 500 ml and a peak airway pressure of 15 cm H_2O:

$$EDC \frac{500 \text{ ml}}{15 \text{ cm } H_2O} = 34 \text{ ml/cm } H_2O$$

The peak airway pressure can be taken from the manometer on the ventilator or using the positive side of a Boehringer inspiratory force manometer. As the patient inhales, a peak is reached at the highest positive inspiratory pressure, for example, 15 to 20 cm H_2O. The normal values for the adult male for EDC are between 40 and 50 ml/cm H_2O and for females between 35 and 45 ml/cm H_2O.

Studies have revealed that as dead space–to–tidal volume ratios are increased, effective compliance falls, which is an indicator that the patient is deteriorating.

The disadvantage in measuring EDC is that other factors are involved, such as airways resistance and the compliance of the thorax as well as that of the abdomen. Clinically, however, it has the advantage of being a simple test; the values obtained, rather than being absolutely accurate, are important when compared with each other to reflect a change in the patient's condition.

Inspiratory force

The amount of ventilatory reserve a patient has is reflected as the muscular ability to be able to move a volume of air sufficient to maintain adequate ventilation. This can be ascertained by measurement of the vital capacity or the inspiratory force. Negative inspiratory force is also a term used for this test because the measurement is made as the total amount of pressure a patient can exert *below* atmospheric pressure in a period of 20 seconds against an occluded airway. This is accomplished by using an inspiratory force manometer that has a manifold with a hole, which is occluded as the patient inhales. Values should exceed 20 cm H_2O negative pressure.

Inspiratory force is reduced where there is a reduction in respiratory muscle function, either because of reduced compliance or from lack of use because of long-term mechanical ventilation. Respiratory center derangement from drugs or damage can also bring about a reduction in inspiratory force.

Gas analysis

The analysis of gases in arterial blood, mixed venous blood, alveolar air, expired air, and inspired air are all important in monitoring respiratory function. Depending on the values obtained from gas analysis, ventilator settings may be altered, inspired oxygen concentrations may be increased or decreased, a patient may be intubated or extubated, and so on.

Respiratory quotient. At the alveolar level, oxygen is removed by hemoglobin while carbon dioxide is unloaded from plasma and hemoglobin. The ratio of carbon dioxide output to the amount of oxygen uptake is known as the respiratory quotient (exchange ratio) and is called R. This ratio is expressed as follows:

$$R = \frac{CO_2 \text{ output ml/min} = 200}{O_2 \text{ uptake ml/min} = 250} = 0.8$$

In most instances gases at the alveolar level are in equilibrium with those in arterial blood. This is more so with carbon dioxide than oxygen because of the small percentage of venous admixture that occurs normally.

Alveolar air equation. A common and valuable method for monitoring the efficiency of oxygen exchange and therapy is to calculate the alveolar-arterial oxygen tension difference (A-aDO$_2$). Normally in persons breathing room air the difference between alveolar and arterial oxygen levels is small (5 to 10 mm Hg). But this difference does increase with age, and in older patients it may be as high as 30 mm Hg.

The alveolar air equation is used to determine A-aDO$_2$ and, in a simple form, may be written as follows:

$$\text{Alveolar } P_{O_2} = \text{Inspired } P_{O_2} - (\text{Arterial } P_{CO_2} \times 1.25)$$

A correction factor of 1.25 is applied to the arterial P_{CO_2} to take into account the respiratory exchange ratio of 0.8. As an illustration, take the example of a person with an inspired oxygen concentration of 150 mm Hg ($F_{I_{O_2}}$ 0.21) and a normal arterial carbon dioxide level of 40 mm Hg:

$$\begin{aligned}
\text{Alveolar } P_{O_2} &= 150 - (40 \times 1.25) \\
&= 150 - 50 \\
&= 100 \text{ mm Hg}
\end{aligned}$$

An alveolar P_{O_2} of 100 mm Hg would normally provide an arterial P_{O_2} of 95 to 100 mm Hg. If, however, the arterial P_{O_2} in this case was found to be only 60 mm Hg, this value deducted from the alveolar P_{O_2} shows an A-aDO$_2$ of 40 mm Hg.

A widening of the alveolar-arterial oxygen tension difference is seen frequently in patients with respiratory failure. Hypoxemia from ventilation- perfusion imbalance, alveolar hypoventilation, physiologic shunts, or diffusion defects (Chapter 8) will result in an increase in A-aDO$_2$.

When interpreting blood gas results, it is extremely important that nurses know what the expected alveolar P_{O_2} should be for a given oxygen concentration and then be able to calculate the A-aDO$_2$. This is a highly sensitive index of oxygen exchange. For example, a patient is receiving 50% oxygen, his arterial blood gas results show a Pa_{O_2} of 110 mm Hg and an arterial P_{CO_2} of 50 mm Hg. Calculate the inspired oxygen concentration and then the alveolar-arterial oxygen tension difference:

$$P_{I_{O_2}} = \frac{50}{100} \times (760 - 47) = 357 \text{ mm Hg}$$

$$\begin{aligned}
\text{Alveolar } P_{O_2} &= P_{I_{O_2}} \ 357 - (P_{a{CO_2}} \ 50 \times 1.25) \\
&= \qquad 62 \\
&= \qquad 295
\end{aligned}$$

Deducting the arterial P_{O_2} 110 mm Hg from the alveolar P_{O_2} of 295 mm Hg, we see an A-aDO$_2$ of 185 mm Hg. This would indicate a large amount of venous admixture or that the inspired oxygen was lower than the stated 50% or that the laboratory was in error.

Arterial blood gas analysis. Measurement of arterial blood gases is now essential to management of the critically ill patient and particularly to those undergoing mechanical ventilation. There are no hard and fast rules applied to the frequency of measurements, which depend on the patient's condition, but certain recommendations have been established. Blood gases should be analyzed as follows:

1. At least once a day for a patient undergoing mechanical ventilation and more frequently during the period of weaning
2. Before and after any changes in ventilator settings or levels of inspired oxygen concentration
3. During any periods when unexpected or unexplained changes in a patient's clinical status occur (Such changes may be reflected as signs and symptoms of hypoxia, hypercapnia, or changes in ventilatory patterns.)

A systematic approach to the interpretation of arterial blood gas measurements is valuable as an aid to assessing the abnormality and to understanding the rationale for therapy. One such method is presented below.

Questions to be considered when evaluating blood gas values:

1. Was it an arterial sample?
2. Was the patient receiving oxygen? If so, how much and by what method?
3. What is the patient's diagnosis?
4. Are we adding to or removing anything from the patient that may alter normal values?
5. What is the patient's fluid and electrolyte status?
6. Are the results believable?

Other important considerations when evaluating blood gas values include looking at each blood gas parameter carefully with respect to the patient's history, present diagnosis, and fluid and electrolyte status and noting indicators for nursing intervention. For example, look for causes of hyperventilation (pain or anxiety) or hypoventilation (sedation or a surgical incision). Note whether the patient is losing acid, for example, from a nasogastric tube, or is increasing hydrogen ion concentration from the accumulation of fixed acids such as ketoacid or lactic acid. Perhaps the patient needs more or less sodium bicarbonate or adjustment in potassium or chloride administration. Check to see whether the patient should be receiving more or less oxygen, and note any treatable causes of shunting such as atelectasis.

Techniques for sampling arterial blood are described in Chapter 5 along with the factors that result in blood gas abnormalities. Some other important things to remember when looking at a blood gas result are that (1) the sum of the arterial PO_2 and the arterial PCO_2 can never be higher than 150 mm Hg in a patient breathing room air at sea level, (2) the relationship between arterial carbon dioxide and alveolar ventilation is almost linear, and (3) an acute rise in arterial carbon dioxide for each 10 mm Hg will bring about a corresponding increase of 1 mEq of bicarbonate.

Mixed venous blood analysis. The reason that mixed venous blood is drawn for analysis is to measure the arteriovenous oxygen difference, either in terms of saturation or oxygen content. Mixed venous blood can also be used for gross cardiac output measurements.

Samples of mixed venous blood may be obtained from a central venous pressure line or more accurately from a pulmonary artery catheter. True mixing of venous blood has occurred only by the time it reaches the pulmonary artery, whereas blood from the superior vena cava does not represent all the venous blood returning to the heart but will serve as a rough guide.

Normally the arteriovenous oxygen difference (a-vO_2) is 4.5 to 5 vol% (arterial 19.7 vol% − venous 15.2 vol%). You will recall that content is dependent on the partial pressure of oxygen to which it is exposed and the amount of available hemoglobin. For example, a venous PO_2 of 40 mm Hg with a saturation of 75% and a hemoglobin of 15 Gm will have an oxygen content of 15.2 vol%. By reducing the hemoglobin to 10 Gm and keeping all other values the same, the content would be 10.2 vol%.

If the oxygen content of mixed venous blood is greatly reduced, there is a widening of the arteriovenous oxygen difference, which means that there has been more oxygen extracted by the tissues. This may be because of tissue hypoxia from a low PO_2, or a reduction in cardiac output, or an increase in oxygen consumption.

In some facilities the oxygen saturation of mixed venous blood is measured routinely at the bedside with the use of an oximeter. The mixed venous PO_2 (Pv_{O_2}) can also be measured and the saturation calculated either using the oxyhemoglobin dissociation curve or a special slide rule designed for that purpose.

CARE OF PATIENTS UNDERGOING MECHANICAL VENTILATION

In critical care settings, such as respiratory intensive care units, coronary care units, and general intensive care units, many patients undergo mechanically assisted ventilation. This places further demands on a nurse's technical and professional skills. Patients may require mechanical ventilation on a short-term basis (for example, for 48 hours postoperatively) or for an extended period of time (weeks or months). Whatever the length of time, certain general considerations apply to management.

Psychological support

An important element for the care of patients undergoing mechanical ventilation is psychological support. The majority of these patients are alert and experience feelings of frustration, anxiety, anger, dependency, denial, and a sense of hopelessness. During periods of intensive respiratory care, a patient's days and nights all run into each other. Schedules are often exhausting, with endless rituals of monitoring vital signs, suctioning, turning, coughing, x-rays, blood work, and so on.

Emotional stress has a marked effect on respiration and can be most troublesome to the patient undergoing mechanical ventilation or to someone who is experiencing respiratory difficulties. The respiratory system is used to express a variety of feelings —laughing, crying, sobbing, singing, sighing—which are most difficult or impossible to express when the patient is being ventilated because of loss of glottic and laryngeal function. Anger causes hyperventilation and often breath-holding. Suppression of anger may result in dyspnea.

Much can be done to help a patient overcome uncomfortable feelings and alleviate stress by controlling the environment. Noise should be kept to a minimum. Remember that the patient usually is subject to the clicking of monitors, clanking of ventilators, and bubbling of chest drainage systems, in addition to the human interaction around him. Nursing a patient in a separate room helps immensely, but when this is not possible, nurses should do everything within their power to reduce noise.

The elements of psychosocial rehabilitation discussed in Chapter 9 should all be applied to the patient undergoing mechanical ventilation: a signal system within easy reach; orientation to time and place; orientation to surroundings, equipment, and function; explanation of procedures; family support; adequate rest; and relief of fears and anxiety. Nurses involved in caring for patients undergoing mechanical ventilation soon become sensitive to the psychological needs of their patients. They recognize that patients need to feel constant reassurance about their progress. They need to feel that their nurses, doctors, and threrapists are capable of taking care of them and handling the equipment. Patients above all need to feel that somebody cares about them.

Physical comfort is an essential element of psychological support. This includes a clean, dry, comfortable bed (an air mattress for the emaciated patient), skin care, mouth care, relief of pain, and careful planning of treatment schedules so that turning and chest physiotherapy and suctioning are coordinated to allow the patient frequent rest periods. When repeated arterial punctures are required, an indwelling catheter to reduce the number of sticks is desirable,

Prevention of complications

Hazards of mechanical ventilation include infection, tracheal trauma, and accidents with the equipment. Infection control includes all the methods and treatments described for the prevention and treatment of respiratory complications. Tracheal trauma is avoided with safe suctioning techniques, proper cuff control (no over-inflation and regular deflation), correct positioning and fixation of the endotracheal or tracheostomy tube, and the use of lightweight tubing, connectors, and swivel adaptors to prevent tube "drag" and to allow the patient movement. Regular tube changes are also recommended to prevent tracheal trauma (at least once each week or when any abnormality in tube or cuff function is suspected).

A mechanical ventilator is a life-support system, and few patients will ever completely overcome the sheer terror experienced if a ventilator fails or they become disconnected from the machine. The patient should be in complete view of an attendant at all times and have some means of summoning help. This is most essential when a patient is paralyzed. In most instances these patients are receiving controlled ventilation on a volume ventilator, which will sound the same whether the patient is connected to it or not. Ventilators equipped with alarm systems greatly reduce the dangerous consequences of such mishaps.

Hand ventilating bags with adaptors should always be at the bedside of patients undergoing mechanical ventilation to provide ventilation should mechanical or electrical power fail.

Weaning

When a patient's ventilatory status is improved sufficiently, the decision is usually made to wean the patient gradually from mechanical ventilation. Nurses and therapists play an important role in helping the patient make a successful transition from the ventilator to spontaneous respiration. Patients often experience feelings of terror during weaning because of the tremendous dependency on "their" machines. This necessitates a gradual weaning process, with careful monitoring to ascertain each patient's ability to breathe without the ventilator or with the use of intermittent mandatory ventilation (IMV) or intermittent demand ventilation (IDV) (p. 154).

Before weaning is attempted, arterial blood gases should be drawn, and vital capacity, tidal volume, and inspiratory force should be measured. Vital capacity should be 15 ml/kg of body weight and the inspiratory force >20 to 30 cm H_2O. During early weaning the nursing staff should stand at the patient's side to reassure constantly, to aspirate secretions when necessary, and to look for signs of fatigue and distress. A physiotherapist who has worked with the patient can greatly assist in continuing to make the patient aware of his respiratory movements.

The effects of emotional stress on respiration should be kept in mind. If the patient is upset or agitated, this will slow progress. Careful attention to the time a patient is supposed to be off the machine is an important factor. Nurses should make sure that the patient is informed of the length of time he is to be tried each session. This period should not be overextended. Setbacks in the weaning process most commonly result from a patient being off the machine for longer periods than ordered; the patient becomes distressed and exhausted and is reluctant to come off the machine for the next session. It is recommended that the patient not be left off the ventilator at night until he has had two consecutive days of spontaneous breathing.

Vital signs monitored during weaning include pulse, blood pressure, tidal volume, breathing frequency, and minute ventilation. (It is advisable to maintain cardiac monitoring during the weaning period for early detection of arrhythmias.) Blood pressure, pulse, and respiratory rate should be monitored at a 5-minute intervals during the first 30 minutes of a weaning session. If the rise in blood pressure is greater than 20 mm Hg, the pulse rate increases to 120 beats a minute, the respiratory rate is greater than 30 breaths a minute, or if the patient becomes anxious, it is recommended that the patient be put back on the ventilator. At the end of 30 minutes if the vital signs are stable, arterial blood gases should be checked and the vital capacity measured.

Apart from the immediate parameters to be monitored before weaning, such as vital capacity, there are certain general physiologic parameters that must be evaluated and corrected before weaning is attempted. These include conditions that affect oxygen transport, consumption, and delivery: fluid, electrolyte, and acid-base abnormalities and the patient's general mental and physical status.

The nurse will recall the factors that affect oxygen transport, such as anemia, reduced cardiac output, and arrhythmias; also the factors affecting oxygen consumption, for example, fever and infection. Fluid, electrolyte, and acid-base abnormalities should also be corrected before weaning.

Metabolic acidosis from hypoxia or a circulatory defect may become worse during weaning, as may hypoventilation, both as a compensatory mechanism of metabolic alkalosis and as a causative condition of respiratory acidosis.

HEMODYNAMIC MONITORING TECHNIQUES*

A high incidence of cardiac arrhythmias occurring in patients undergoing mechanical ventilation has been reported in many studies. This is partly due to the effects of mechanical ventilation on cardiorespiratory function and the effects of hypoxia and acidosis on circulatory function. Continuous cardiac monitoring is recommended with an oscilloscope that provides an instant rhythm strip when required.

Frequent measurements (hourly or less initially) of blood pressure and apical and radial pulses are required. Signs of hypoxia may first become apparent with sudden hypertension, tachycardia, or cardiac arrhythmias; impending circulatory failure is also frequently secondary to hypoxia. Other parameters to assess a patient's hemodynamic and cardiopulmonary status particularly are measurements of central venous pressure, pulmonary artery pressure, and pulmonary artery wedge pressure.

Central venous pressure (CVP)

Central venous pressure refers to the blood pressure in the great veins of the thorax and is usually measured in the superior vena cava. It reflects the pressure in the right atrium and the diastolic filling pressure of the right ventricle. The CVP is determined by blood volume, vascular tone, and cardiac contractility. Thus the CVP represents the relationship between circulating blood volume and the competency of the heart to handle that volume at that particular time. When the heart is pumping adequately, the CVP varies *directly* with changes in blood volume. When the blood volume and vascular dynamics are adequate and stable, the CVP varies *inversely* with cardiac compliance and with cardiac contractility.

As a measurement of the filling pressure of the right side of the heart, CVP monitoring is useful in assessing blood volume and adequacy of venous return. This information is particularly important in caring for postoperative patients or patients with hypovolemia or hypervolemia. The value of the information in monitoring patients with cardiopulmonary disease is mainly as an index of the performance of the right side of the heart. It is also useful in monitoring blood volume (venous return) and provides an intravenous line for administering a fluid challenge and for sampling venous blood. When pulmonary artery (PA) monitoring is not possible, the CVP is sometimes used as a relative guide in assessing left heart pressures. This is a poor guide because left heart pressure changes are unpredictably transmitted through the capillary bed to the right side of the heart. Although failure of the left ventricle will eventually cause a rise in the CVP, this usually occurs only after the right heart has failed as well.

The normal CVP is 4 to 8 cm H_2O. Low pressures may be seen in patients with hypovolemia from a variety of causes. Pressures higher than 8 cm H_2O are seen in patients with hypervolemia, cardiac tamponade, constrictive pericardial disease, or cardiac failure. Errors in misinterpretation of CVP values can be reduced by careful correlation of pressure readings with the overall clinical situation.

---

*Written by Elaine Kiess Daily, R.N., R.C.V.T., Cardiovascular Nurse Specialist, Stanford University Medical Center, Stanford, Calif.

The value of measuring central venous pressure has been questioned in many instances, but present data support CVP measurements during fluid resuscitation using the fluid challenge routine. For example, a baseline CVP is obtained, and fluid is administered in either 50, 100, or 200 ml over a 10-minute period. After 10 minutes a second CVP measurement is taken, and if the CVP has increased by 2 cm H_2O or less, a second fluid challenge is administered over another 10 minutes. The central venous pressure is then measured again, and if the pressure increase exceeds 2 cm H_2O but is 5 cm H_2O or less, the procedure is stopped for 10 minutes in order to wait to reevaluate the patient's status. If at the end of the 10-minute period the CVP has decreased to within 2 cm H_2O of the value prior to the last fluid challenge, then the procedure is continued. A fluid challenge routine is stopped if either the CVP rises 5 cm H_2O or more during any one challenge or if the pressure does not return to within 2 cm H_2O of the previous challenge period.

Some recent studies indicate that a rise in CVP occurring simultaneously with a fall in systemic blood pressure provides a valuable index for early recognition of cardiac tamponade.

Respiratory variation is frequently noted in CVP tracings with a drop in pressure occurring during normal inspiration because of the changes in intrathoracic pressure. Mechanical ventilation causes an increase in central venous pressure because of increases in intrathoracic pressure. PEEP and all its variants also bring about an increase in CVP.

As with all pressure monitoring, a single CVP reading is of less value than serial measurements, which are necessary to reflect the trend of the venous pressure and evaluate the response to therapy.

Pulmonary artery pressure (PA)

Overall cardiac function is best determined by the performance of the main pumping chamber of the heart, the left ventricle (LV). Left ventricular performance, in turn, is primarily determined by the left ventricular end-diastolic pressure (LVedp) according to the Frank-Starling ventricular-function curve. The end-diastolic or filling pressure is the pressure required for the left ventricle to fill with blood adequately. It is determined by the initial stretch of the myocardial fibers at end-diastole and reflects the compliance of the left ventricle. In the compliant, nondiseased ventricle, the end-diastolic pressure is low (5 to 12 mm Hg). A damaged or poorly functioning left ventricle is not compliant and is stiff and resistant to filling. Thus a higher end-diastolic pressure is required to allow sufficient filling to maintain adequate stroke volume (the amount of blood ejected by the ventricle with each heartbeat). Direct measurement of LVedp through the use of a catheter in the left ventricle is a complex procedure confined to the diagnostic cardiac catheterization laboratory. Bedside, indirect monitoring of left ventricular function is available, however, with the use of the flow-directed, balloon-tipped catheter. This catheter allows direct measurement of both pulmonary artery (PA) and pulmonary artery wedge (PAW) pressures, which are an indirect measurement of LVedp.

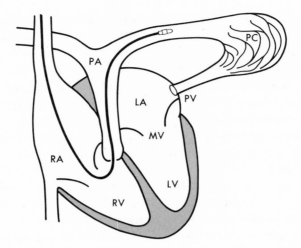

FIG. 11-2. Anatomic illustration of left ventricular, *LV*, end-diastole showing the mitral valve open and the left ventricle filled with blood just prior to atrial systole. At this point there is equalization of pressures between the left ventricle, *LV*; left atrium, *LA*; pulmonary veins, *PV*; pulmonary capillaries, *PC*; and pulmonary artery, *PA*. *RA*, Right atrium; *RV*, right ventricle; *MV*, mitral value.

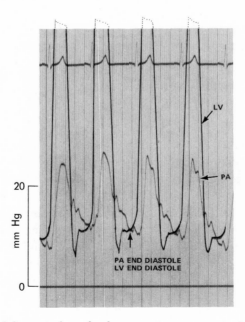

FIG. 11-3. Simultaneous left ventricular and pulmonary artery pressure tracing. Note the close correlation between *LV* and *PA* end-diastole: *PA* systolic pressure = 29 mm Hg; diastolic pressure = 12 mm Hg. *LV* systolic pressure is off scale; diastolic pressure = 12 mm Hg. The dark vertical time lines are 1 second apart; the light lines mark every 0.2 second. (From Schroeder, J. S., and Daily, E. K.: Techniques in bedside hemodynamic monitoring, St. Louis, 1976, The C. V. Mosby Co.)

The PA pressure is divided into two phases: systole and diastole. The systolic pressure is the peak pressure generated by the right ventricle. The diastolic pressure is the lowest pressure in the PA and occurs just prior to the next right ventricular systole. Fig. 11-2 is an anatomic illustration of end-diastole and shows the relation of the LVedp to the PA end-diastolic pressure. Just before atrial systole, at the end of diastole, the mitral valve is open, and the left ventricle is filled with blood. At this point there is an equalization of pressures between the left ventricle, and left atrium (if there is no mitral valve disease), the pulmonary veins, the pulmonary capillaries, and the pulmonary artery. Therefore the end-diastolic pressure of the PA equals the end-diastolic pressure of the left ventricle and can be used to monitor accurately LVedp and left ventricular function. Fig. 11-3 shows the close correlation between the LV and PA end-diastolic pressures.

Fig. 11-4 is an illustration of the PA wave form showing a steep rise during right ventricular systole after the pulmonic valve has opened. This is the systolic pressure of the PA and is followed by diastole, manifested by a gradual decrease in pressure during ejection of blood from the right ventricle into the PA. The sudden closure of the pulmonic valve causes a momentary rise in pressure and is seen as the dicrotic notch. Thereafter the pressure continues to fall until the next systole occurs. The period just prior to the next systole is termed the *end-diastolic pressure*.

PA systolic pressure is normally 20 to 30 mm Hg, and diastolic pressure is <10

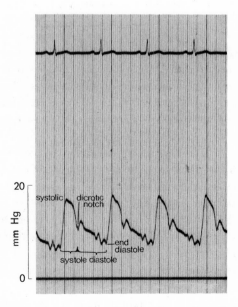

FIG. 11-4. Pulmonary artery pressure wave form showing phases of systole, dicrotic notch (pulmonary valve closure), and diastole. Normally, pulmonary diastole closely represents LVedp. (From Schroeder, J. S., and Daily, E. K.: Techniques in bedside hemodynamic monitoring, St. Louis, 1976, The C. V. Mosby Co.)

mm Hg. PA mean pressure is an average of the systolic and diastolic pressures and is normally <20 mm Hg.

Respiratory variation also may be noted in PA pressure tracings due to changes in intrathoracic pressure. Having the patient breathe quietly during the pressure measurement minimizes this problem.

The PA pressure is abnormally elevated in patients receiving positive pressure ventilation as a result of a significant increase in pulmonary vascular resistance. This pressure increase will subside, however, when the patient is removed from the ventilator. If possible, therefore, positive pressure ventilation should be removed when measuring PA pressure. But it is more important to establish a consistent pattern of measuring pressures, with the patient either on or preferably off the ventilator. As with the CVP, reliance should not be placed on any single pressure reading. Serial pressure measurements are necessary to reveal the trend of PA pressure changes.

Other causes of elevated PA pressures include (1) pulmonary vascular disease, (2) mitral valve disease, (3) pulmonary embolism, (4) left ventricular failure, (5) constrictive pericardial disease, and (6) hypoxia.

Pulmonary artery wedge pressure (PAW)

The PAW pressure is the pressure measurement obtained when a catheter is "wedged" tightly in a small branch of pulmonary artery, allowing the measurement of pressure beyond the tip of the catheter in the more distal pulmonary capillaries and pulmonary veins. It is more accurately termed pulmonary capillary pressure. This pressure is essentially the same as the left atrial pressure and the filling pressure of the left ventricle (LVedp). As mentioned and illustrated previously, at left ventricular end-diastole there is equilibration of pressures back to the PA. For this reason the mean PAW pressure is also an accurate reflection of LVedp in the absence of mitral valve disease and can be used to monitor left ventricular function. Fig. 11-5 demonstrates the correlation between PAW and LV end-diastolic pressures.

Fig. 11-6 is an illustration of the PAW pressure wave form, showing its similarity to an atrial pressure tracing. The PAW pressure wave consists of three waves: the *a* wave, the *c* wave, and the *v* wave. The *a* wave is a distinct wave that is produced by the rise in atrial pressure during left atrial systole. In actual timing, it occurs with the P wave of the electrocardiogram. On recordings, however, it occurs slightly after the P wave because of the time delay from the pressure event to the transducer. The *c* wave is a small and frequently nonvisible pressure change that occurs during closure of the mitral valve. The *v* wave is a distinct wave produced by the increase in left atrial pressure that occurs when the mitral valve bulges back into the atrium during left ventricular systole. In actual timing the *v* wave occurs with the T wave of the electrocardiogram. Again, there is a slight delay noted in recordings. The descent of the *a* wave is termed the *x* descent, and the descent of the *v* wave is the *y* descent.

The mean PAW pressure is normally between 4 and 12 mm Hg. As with the CVP and PA pressures, significant respiratory variation may occur in the PAW pressure

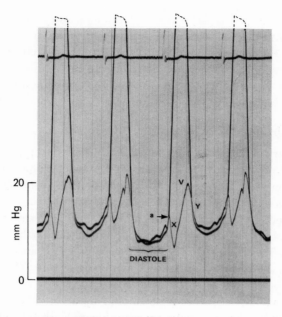

FIG. 11-5. Simultaneous recording of left ventricular and pulmonary artery wedge pressures. Note the normal *a* and *v* waves with *x* and *y* descents. During diastole, the PAW pressure is barely 1 mm higher than the left ventricular pressure when the mitral valve is open and blood is flowing from the left atrium to the left ventricle. (From Schroeder, J. S., and Daily, E. K.: Techniques in bedside hemodynamic monitoring, St. Louis, 1976, The C. V. Mosby Co.)

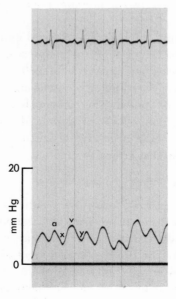

FIG. 11-6. Normal pulmonary artery wedge pressure tracing showing *a* and *v* waves and *x* and *y* descents.

tracing. An increase in pulmonary vascular resistance and elevated PAW pressures are usually seen with the use of positive pressure ventilation. Serial pressure measurements should always be taken consistently, with the patient either on or off the ventilator, to determine any hemodynamic changes.

Other causes of elevated PAW pressures include (1) pulmonary vascular disease, (2) mitral valve disease, and (3) left ventricular failure.

PA and PAW catheters

Fig. 11-7 illustrates one type of flow-directed, balloon-tipped catheter used to monitor PA and PAW pressures. This catheter has two lumens: one for inflation of the balloon and one for pressure measurement or fluid administration. A triple-lumen catheter has a third lumen, which terminates 20 to 30 cm proximal to the tip, allowing simultaneous pressure measurements of the CVP and PA or for the administration of fluid. A quadruple-lumen catheter has a fourth lumen, which contains a thermistor. This catheter is used for thermodilution cardiac output measurements. Pulmonary artery catheters are available in 5F, 6F, or 7F and are 100 cm in length.

The catheter may be introduced into a vein by a cutdown, or percutaneously using a needle, guide wire, and catheter introducer. With the catheter connected to a transducer and monitoring system, the catheter is advanced to the right atrium. The balloon is then inflated with the appropriate amount of gas (either air or carbon dioxide) and, with continuous monitoring, allowed to advance with the flow of blood to the PA. Fig. 11-8 shows an example of the type of pressure tracings obtained as the catheter advances through each chamber of the heart. When the catheter tip has reached the PA (as documented by the pressure tracing), the balloon is deflated and advanced slightly.

To obtain a PAW pressure, the balloon is inflated until there is a distinct change in the wave form (Fig. 11-9). The principle of this pressure measurement is the same as that of tightly wedging the catheter in a small branch of the pulmonary artery. With the balloon inflated, the tip of the catheter is measuring the pressure distal to it, that is, in the pulmonary capillary system. The balloon should be inflated only with the amount of air necessary to obtain a PAW pressure and only for brief periods of time, because prolonged blockage of the artery by the balloon can cause an infarction to the area of the lung supplied by that artery.

PA catheter complications

Passage of the flow-directed, balloon-tipped catheter may produce either atrial or ventricular arrhythmias because of mechanical irritation produced by the catheter. These arrhythmias are usually transient and disappear completely once the catheter is situated well into the PA. The sudden development of arrhythmias after catheter placement in the PA could indicate migration of the catheter back into the right ventricle or even the right atrium. This can be documented by the corresponding pressure tracing and corrected by repositioning the catheter.

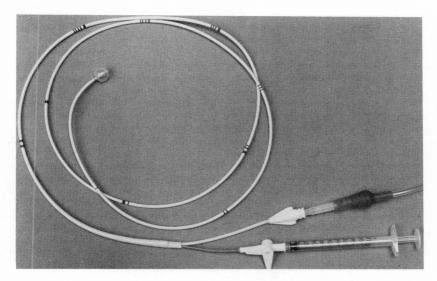

FIG. 11-7. Swan-Ganz flow-directed, balloon-tipped catheter for pulmonary artery pressure monitoring. The tuberculin syringe is used for inflating the balloon with air. Intravenous tubing is attached to the other lumen for infusion of fluid or pressure measurement at the catheter tip. (From Schroeder, J. S., and Daily, E. K.: Techniques in bedside hemodynamic monitoring, St. Louis, 1976, The C. V. Mosby Co.)

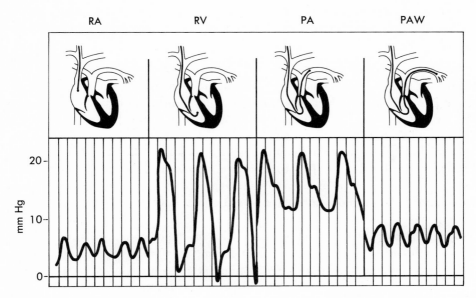

FIG. 11-8. Flow-directed balloon tipped catheter positions with corresponding pressure tracings. *RA*, right atrium; *RV*, right ventricle; *PA*, pulmonary artery; and *PAW*, pulmonary artery wedge.

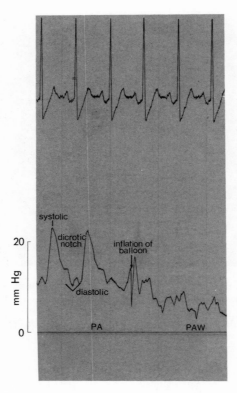

FIG. 11-9. Pulmonary artery pressure wave form via a balloon-tipped catheter. Note the balloon inflation and the subsequent change to a pulmonary artery wedge pressure wave form. (From Schroeder, J. S., and Daily, E. K.: Techniques in bedside hemodynamic monitoring, St. Louis, 1976, The C. V. Mosby Co.)

Rupture of the balloon of the catheter can occur and should be suspected when injection of air into the balloon fails to produce a feeling of resistance or fails to produce a PAW tracing. No further attempts should be made to inflate the balloon or obtain a PAW pressure. The PA diastolic pressure can continue to be used, however, to monitor left ventricular function.

Thrombus formation at the tip of the catheter poses a serious problem in the use of balloon-tipped catheters. This complication should be suspected when pressure tracings are damped or flat or when the intravenous drip is not infusing well. The use of heparinized intravenous fluid and a continuous flow device may prevent this problem.

By far the most serious complication of balloon-tipped catheters is the development of pulmonary hemorrhage or infarction, and it is frequently indicated by the sudden development of hemoptysis. This complication is caused by overinflation of the balloon while the catheter is wedged or by prolonged inflation of the balloon. Inflating the balloon with only the amount of air necessary to obtain a PAW pressure for extremely brief periods of time can prevent the development of this complication.

Although the CVP is a reliable index of the performance of the right side of the heart, it does not always correlate with hemodynamic changes in the left side of the heart. This is particularly true in patients with acute myocardial infarction and failure of the left ventricle. More direct measurement and monitoring of left ventricular pressure and function are desirable in caring for these critically ill patients. The flow-directed, balloon-tipped catheter can be inserted at the bedside and allows long-term monitoring of either PA diastolic or mean PAW pressures indicating left atrial and left ventricular diastolic filling pressures. These parameters provide data necessary to evaluate left ventricular function and vascular volume and are vital in monitoring the unstable cardiopulmonary patient with rapidly changing hemodynamics.

MISCELLANEOUS MONITORING
Oxygen therapy

Techniques for measuring the effectiveness of oxygen therapy include measurements of arterial Po_2 (on room air and 50% or 100% oxygen), $A-aDo_2$, mixed venous Po_2, P_{50}, and inspired oxygen concentrations. Measurements of ventilation, hemoglobin concentration, and cardiac output are also important in terms of oxygen uptake, transport, and delivery.

Accurate determinations of the fractional inspired oxygen concentration (FI_{O_2}) are essential when evaluating the effectiveness of oxygen therapy. This can be done with oxygen analyzers and by knowing the percentage of oxygen delivered by various pieces of equipment at different flow rates. Before an arterial blood sample is drawn and analyzed, the patient should remain on the specified amount of oxygen for at least 10 minutes. The amount of oxygen being administered as well as the method being used should be clearly indicated on the patient's flow sheet and laboratory requisition at the time the sample is to be drawn. Arterial blood gas measurements are costly to a patient, and every effort to maintain bedside quality control is advisable.

Because venous–to–arterial shunting is so common to the critically ill patient, it is highly desirable to evaluate the degree of shunting present in a patient and to select an appropriate inspired oxygen concentration that will provide an adequate Po_2 in that patient. Graphic aids for this purpose have been developed and are called iso-shunt graphs (Fig. 11-10).

The graph was constructed taking into account several physiologic parameters that affect oxygen uptake and transport, such as cardiac output, physiologic shunting, arterio-mixed venous oxygen content difference, hemoglobin, and factors that shift the oxyhemoglobin dissociation curve. The graph presented in Fig. 11-10 shows shunt lines constructed within a range of 10 to 14 Gm of hemoglobin, a $PaCO_2$ of 25 to 40 mm Hg, and a normal arterio-mixed venous oxygen content difference of 5 vol%. Dr. S. R. Benatar and his colleagues use the term *virtual shunt* for the shunt value obtained when using the graph to indicate the arteriovenous oxygen content difference of 5 vol%.

To use the graph the arterial Po_2 of a patient is measured at a given FI_{O_2}. The

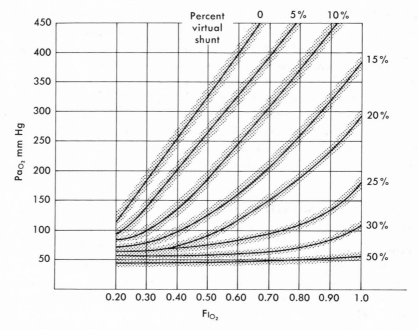

FIG. 11-10. Iso-shunt lines for control of oxygen therapy. (See text for description.) (From Benatar, S. R., Hewlett, A. M., and Nunn, J. F.: Brit. J. Anaesth. **45:**711-718, 1973.)

result is then plotted on the graph to derive the virtual shunt. The iso-shunt line is then followed down to a point that a desired Pa_{O_2} is indicated, and the $F_{I_{O_2}}$ that will provide that Po_2 is then read off the vertical axis. For example, a patient is receiving 70% oxygen, and the arterial Po_2 is found to be 200 mm Hg: This would give a virtual shunt value of 15%. If this line is then followed down to a point where it matches a desired arterial Po_2 of 110 mm Hg, the $F_{I_{O_2}}$ that will provide this (45%) can be read off the horizontal axis.

The iso-shunt line graph is most useful for predicting the $F_{I_{O_2}}$ at which an optimal Po_2 can be obtained and thus reduces the number of arterial blood gases required to control oxygen therapy.

Computerized monitoring

With advances in technology, computer-based bedside monitoring of patients in critical care settings has proved to be of great value in providing continuous measurements of the cardiopulmonary system. Some medical centers have units where recorded measurements are seen at each bedside on the computer terminals as whole numbers or as a wave form plot. Recorded data are available at particular time intervals (such as every 10 minutes) or on demand and as a permanent printout for the patient's chart at the end of the shift. With the use of a simple keyboard, a variety of patient information can be retrieved quickly; or data such as the patient's name, age, height, weight, or laboratory results can be entered into the system.

When employed with a flow-sensing device, a computerized monitoring system can be used to measure a number of parameters of respiratory function, for example, tidal volume, minute volume, end tidal P_{CO_2}, flow rates, pressure-volume curves, and alveolar oxygen concentrations.

REFERENCES

Adams, N. R.: Reducing the perils of intracardiac monitoring, Nursing **76**(4):66-75, 1976.

Benatar, S. R., Hewlett, A. M., and Nunn, J. F.: The use of iso-short lines for control of oxygen therapy, Br. J. Anaesth. **45**:711-719, 1973.

Bushnell, S. S.: Respiratory intensive care nursing, Boston, 1973, Little, Brown & Co.

Downs, J. B., Klein, E. F., Desautels, D., Modell, J. H., and Kirby, R.: Intermittent mandatory ventilation: a new approach to weaning patients from mechanical ventilation, Chest **64**:331-335, 1973.

Fitzgerald, L. M., and Huber, G. L.: Weaning the patient from mechanical ventilation, Heart Lung **5**:228-234, 1976.

Hodgkin, J. E., Bowser, M. A., and Burton, G. G.: Respirator weaning, Crit. Care Med. **2**:95-103, 1974.

Martz, K. V., and Beaumont, J. O.: Computer-based monitoring in an intensive care unit (ICU); implication for nursing education, Heart Lung **1**:90-99, 1972.

Osborn, J.: Monitoring respiratory junction, Crit. Care Med. **4**:217-221, 1974.

Qvist, J., Pontoppidan, H., Wilson, R. S., Lowenstien, E., and Laver, M. B.: Hemodynamic responses to mechanical ventilation with PEEP, Anesthesiology **42**:45-55, 1975.

Rushmer, R. F.: Structure and function of the cardiovascular system, Philadelphia, 1972, W. B. Saunders Co.

Rutherford, B. D., McCann, W. D., and O'Donovan, T. P.: The value of monitoring pulmonary artery pressure for early detection of left ventricular failure following myocardial infarction, Circulation **43**:655-665, 1971.

Sahn, S. A., and Lakshminarayan, S.: Bedside criteria for discontinuation of mechanical ventilation, Chest **63**:1002-1005, 1973.

Sarwar, H. A. S., et al.: Pulmonary arterial monitoring in cardiac tamponade (abstract), Fifth Annual Society of Critical Care Medicine Meeting, San Francisco, 1976.

Schroeder, J. S., and Daily, E. K.: Techniques in bedside hemodynamic monitoring, St. Louis, 1976, The C. V. Mosby Co.

Shapiro, B. A., Harrison, R. A., Walton, J. R., and Davidson, R.: Intermittent demand ventilation (IDV): a new technique for supporting ventilation in critically ill patients, Respir. Care **21**:521-525, 1976.

Shapiro, P. M., Friedman, G. K., and Niccotra, M. B.: The value of flow directed intravascular catheters in cardiorespiratory failure, Am. Rev. Respir. Dis. **107**:1111-1112, 1973.

Swan, H. J. C., Ganz, W., Forrester, J. S., Marcus, H., Diamond, G., and Chonette, D.: Catheterization of the heart in man with use of a flow-directed balloon tipped catheter, N. Engl. J. Med. **283**:447-451, 1970.

Vinicur, B., Sheldon, A. J., Sampliner, J. E.: Application of a critical care monitoring program in the diagnosis and management of critically ill patients (abstract), 45th Annual Scientific Assembly of the American College of Chest Physicians, 1975.

Wasserman, K., Selecky, P., and Ziment, I.: A graphical approach to assess $V_E - Pa_{CO_2} - V_D/V_T$ relationships in patients on respirators, Am. Rev. Respir. Dis. (In press.)

Wilson, J. N., Grow, J. B., Demong, C. V., Preveded, A. E., and Owens, J. C.: Central venous pressure in optimal blood volume maintenance, Arch. Surg. **85**:563-578, 1962.

Wilson, R. S., and Pontoppidan, H.: Acute respiratory failure: diagnostic and therapeutic criteria. In Shoemaker, W. C., editor: The lung in the critically ill patient, Baltimore, 1976, The Williams & Wilkins Co.

Zschoche, D., editor: Respiratory concepts, Crit. Care Update, March, 1975.

TERMINOLOGY
Symbols and abbreviations used in respiratory physiology

This listing is based on standardization of definitions and symbols in respiratory physiology, Federation Proc. 9:602-605, 1950. See also newer terms and symbols on p. 215.

GENERAL

- **V** gas volume
- **V̇** gas volume per unit of time
- **P** gas pressure in general
- **Q** volume of blood
- **Q̇** volume flow of blood per unit of time
- **S** percent saturation of hemoglobin with oxygen or carbon monoxide
- **f** breathing frequency

SECONDARY SYMBOLS

Gas phase only

- I inspired gas
- E expired gas
- D dead space gas
- A alveolar gas
- T tidal gas
- L lung
- B barometric

Blood phase only

- **a** arterial
- **v** venous
- **c** capillary

EXAMPLES

Pa_{O_2} partial pressure of oxygen in arterial blood

Pa_{CO_2} partial pressure of carbon dioxide in arterial blood
PA_{O_2} partial pressure of oxygen in alveolar gas
PI_{O_2} partial pressure of oxygen in inspired gas
PB barometric pressure
VT tidal volume
VD volume of dead space
$\dot{V}E$ volume of expired gas per unit of time (minute ventilation)
$\dot{V}A$ volume of alveolar gas per unit of time (alveolar ventilation)

LUNG VOLUMES

VC   vital capacity
IC   inspiratory capacity
IRV   inspiratory reserve volume
ERV   expiratory reserve volume
FRC   functional residual capacity
RV   residual volume
VT   tidal volume
TLC   total lung capacity
-     a dash above any symbol indicates a mean value
·   a dot above any symbol indicates a rate or time derivation

PULMONARY MECHANICS

MEFR   maximal expiratory flow rate
MMFR   maximal mid-flow rate
MIFR   maximal inspiratory flow rate
MVV   maximal voluntary ventilation
FEV   forced expiratory volume

NEWER PULMONARY TERMS AND SYMBOLS*

CV   closing volume
CC   closing capacity
FVC   forced vital capacity (formerly TVC)
FEF200-1200   mean forced expiratory flow between 200 and 1,200 ml (formerly MEFR)
FEC25-75%   mean forced expiratory flow during the middle half of the FVC (formerly MMFR)
$P(A-a)O_2$ alveolar-arterial oxygen pressure difference (formerly A-aDO_2)

---

*Older terms are left in Appendix A because they are still seen extensively in the literature.

HENDERSON-HASSELBALCH EQUATION

One method of calculating the pH of a buffer system is by using the Henderson-Hasselbalch equation. In clinical medicine it may be used to calculate any one of the three parameters of acid-base balance: pH, Pa_{CO_2} or bicarbonate. The equation in clinical form may be written:

$$pH = pK + \log \frac{HCO_3^- \text{ mEq/liter}}{P_{CO_2} \text{ mm Hg} \times 0.03}$$
(6.1)

This form of the equation was derived as follows:

A buffer solution is made up of a weak or poorly ionized acid and its dissociated salt, which tend to minimize changes in hydrogen ion (H^+) concentration when either a strong acid or base is added to the solution.

Thus the equation in an early stage is written as a buffer equation:

$$[H^+] = K_a \frac{[\text{acid}]}{[\text{salt}]}$$

K_a is a dissociation constant that expresses the degree of ionization an acid undergoes. Because the numbers are so small, the K_a of a system is expressed in terms of its negative logarithm, called the pK of a system. pH is also expressed as the negative logarithm of the hydrogen ion concentration. Therefore:

$$(-\log[H^+]) \text{ pH} = pK (-\log K_a) + \left(-\log \frac{[\text{acid}]}{[\text{salt}]} \right)$$

The equation can be changed around and written as follows:

$$pH = pK + \log \frac{[\text{base}]}{[\text{acid}]}$$

In the case of the carbonic acid/bicarbonate system:

$$pH = pK + \log \frac{[HCO_3^-]}{[CO_2]}$$

The carbonic acid dissociation constant is 7.85×10^{-7}, which converts mathematically into a pK of 6.1. As the equation stands, the denominator expresses dissolved carbon dioxide, which is not measured in blood, but the partial pressure of

216

the gas P_{CO_2} is. This is directly proportional to the concentration of dissolved carbon dioxide and may be substituted in the denominator. Therefore, if an arterial P_{CO_2} is 40 mm Hg and a bicarbonate concentration is 24 mEq/liter:

$$pH = 6.1 + \log \frac{24}{1.2} \; (40 \text{ mm Hg} \times 0.03)$$
$$= 6.1 + \log 20$$
$$= 6.1 + 1.30$$
$$= 7.40$$

APPENDIX C

PATTERNS OF RESPIRATION

eupnea The normal spontaneous respiration of which one is usually unaware.

apnea Complete absence or cessation of breathing, which may occur intermittently in patients with central nervous system disturbances or drug intoxication. When the condition persists, it constitutes a respiratory arrest.

dyspnea A subjective sensation of shortness of breath, which is a symptom commonly experienced by patients with pulmonary or cardiac disease. Patients may not feel dyspneic until they exercise, in which case sudden attempts of the body to increase ventilation and cardiac output are partly blocked by the underlying disease process.

orthopnea The feeling of dyspnea experienced by a patient in the recumbent position. It is relieved when the patient assumes the upright position. Conditions such as left ventricular failure and pulmonary edema predispose the symptom.

hyperventilation Overventilation with an increase in the volume of air entering the alveoli greater than required for body metabolism. Alveolar hyperventilation results in hypocapnia.

hypoventilation Underventilation with a decrease in the volume of air entering the alveoli with respect to the metabolic needs of the body. Alveolar hypoventilation always results in hypercapnia and hypoxemia.

tachypnea An increase in breathing frequency that may be associated with either hyperventilation or hypoventilation. Patients with hypoventilation associated with restrictive diseases frequently have tachypnea.

Kussmaul respiration The type of respiration associated with diabetic acidosis, characterized by an abnormal increase in the depth and rate of breathing. This results from a compensatory attempt by the body to restore pH by eliminating carbon dioxide.

hyperpnea A normal increase in ventilation to meet an increase in metabolic demand, for example, during exercise.

Biot's breathing An irregular respiratory pattern both of rate and tidal volume, which is associated with central nervous system disturbances.

Cheyne-Stokes respiration A pattern of periodic breathing characterized by initial shallow respirations, which increase in depth, reach a peak, and decline; a period of apnea follows, then the cycle is repeated. This pattern is maintained by a buildup of carbon dioxide during the period of apnea, which, in its turn, stimulates respiration.

INDEX

A

Aarane; *see* Cromolyn sodium
Absolute humidity, 18
Absolute temperature scale; *see* Kelvin temperature scale
ACCP-ATS Joint Committee on Pulmonary Nomenclature, 28
Acetazolamide, 162
Acetylcysteine, 157
Acid
amino, 61-62
and bases, 64
carbonic, 64
hydrochloric, 64
para-aminosalicylic, 92
Acid-base disturbances
drugs used in treatment of, 161-162
metabolic, 67
possible causes of, 68
respiratory, 67
respiratory and metabolic, 68-71
Acidosis, 50, 57, 64, 69
acute respiratory, 67, 68
chronic respiratory, 67, 68
correction in treatment of status asthmaticus, 182
metabolic, 67, 68, 70-71
respiratory, 68-70
Acinar gas-exchanging unit, 4
Acinus, component parts of, 4
Adenosine diphosphate, 14
3'-5'-Adenosine monophosphate, 87, 157
Adenosine triphosphate, 13, 14, 87, 157
Admixture, venous, 60
ADP; *see* Adenosine diphosphate
Adrenalin; *see* Epinephrine
beta-Adrenergic blockage theory, 87
Adrenergic receptor, 157
ADRS; *see* Respiratory distress syndrome, adult
Adventitious breath sounds, 103
Aerobacter, 156
Aerobic metabolism, 13, 14
Aerosol, 105
corticosteroid, 160
Age
and changes in vital capacity, 32
as predisposing factor to chronic bronchitis and emphysema, 80-81
Ahlquist, R. P., 87
Air, composition of, 17

Air bronchogram sign, 118
"Air hunger," 142-143
Air Shields, 175
Air trapping, 29
Airflow; *see* Flow
Airway
conducting, and uneven distribution of ventilation, 43
oropharyngeal, 144
patency of, 143-151, 171
Airway dysfunction, tests for, 48
Airways resistance, 45, 46
Alkalosis, 57, 64
acute respiratory, 67
chronic respiratory, 67
metabolic, 67, 68, 70, 71
respiratory, 68, 70
Allergen, 86
Altitude, adjustment to, 129
Alupent; *see* Metaproterenol
Alveolar air equation, 197
Alveolar cell, 5, 6
Alveolar dead space, 41
Alveolar duct, 3
Alveolar expansion, 78, 90-91
Alveolar hypoventilation, 42, 68-69, 83, 127
Alveolar macrophage, 5, 11
Alveolar pore, 4
Alveolar sac, 3
Alveolar ventilation, 41-42, 48-49
in chronic obstructive pulmonary disease, 179
Alveolar-capillary membrane, 4-5
Alveolar-lining membranes and cellular function, 4-5
Alveoli, 3-4
layers of, 5
and uneven distribution of ventilation, 43
Ambient temperature, ambient pressure saturated, 21, 22
AMBU, 175
American Heart Association Committee on Cardiopulmonary Resuscitation and Emergency Cardiac Care, 170
American Thoracic Society, 86
Amesec, 160
Amino acid, 61-62
Aminodur Dura-Tabs, 160
Aminophylline, 37, 159, 181-182, 186
Ammonia, 67

219